PRAISE FC

WHOLE MEDICINE

"The psychedelic landscape is quickly evolving. Ms. Martinez provides much needed ethical guidance for both psychedelic facilitators and the folks who want to use them, and she does it with grace and compassion. It's my hope people in the field will consider the careful recommendations in *Whole Medicine*. They couldn't be more timely."

—EUGENIA BONE, author of *Mycophilia* and *Microbia*

"*Whole Medicine* covers the whole relational landscape of therapeutic plant medicines and psychedelics. Rebecca uncovers and beautifully describes the ethos and interrelationships that sustain and balance this ecosystem below its surface. Rebecca articulates the value of inner work, the nuances of presence, the critical importance of compassion, and the conscious use of power, and we come to understand how much we need one another in community. The book is an amazingly comprehensive guide to ethical participation in this field, for whatever role you play within it."

—KYLEA TAYLOR, author of *The Ethics of Caring*

"*Whole Medicine* is an important contribution to the psychedelic landscape at a pivotal time. It is a refreshingly honest and humble approach to psychedelic healing work, making it an integral resource for facilitators, journeyers, and psychedelic companies alike. A must-read for anyone pursuing the psychedelic path that examines all aspects of living a psychedelic life with integrity—without ignoring the challenges the burgeoning new industry and grassroots community face—all told in a compassionate and thought-provoking way."

—MICHELLE JANIKIAN, author of *Your Psilo- cybin Mushroom Companion*

"Rebecca Martinez has created a truly insightful, gentle, and thorough overview of approaches to inner work, reciprocity, sharing of power, consent, and accountability. . . . This seminal volume has evolved from the experiences of the underground therapists, the newcomers, and the Indigenous people who were first to learn of the magic and effectiveness of these healing arts. . . . Vulnerable souls who seek an end to suffering, together with those who attempt to confront and resolve difficulties of heart and mind, will find careful guidance herein."

—WILLIAM LEONARD PICKARD, author of
The Rose of Paracelsus

"*Whole Medicine* is an essential and much-needed contribution to the field. Rebecca's self-awareness throughout the book provides readers with a model of integrity and honesty when navigating the terrain of their own consciousness and the responsibility that comes with holding space for others. Rebecca offers a solid foundation for how to be in and with community as we journey together toward healing and liberation. The guidance offered in *Whole Medicine* is filled with awe and humility. Anyone who has deeply felt inner conflict will resonate with this text, regardless of where they are in the process of regaining balance and wholeness."

—JULIA MANDE, systems change facilitator
and organizational designer

"Discourse around psychedelics too often focuses on the individual and overlooks many relevant current and historical contexts, like the lasting legacy of historical trauma and systemic injustice. *Whole Medicine* invites us deep into multidimensional reflection and delves into layers often missing from our collective conversations."

—JOSEPH McCOWAN, PhD, PsyD, clinical
psychologist, psychedelic therapist, and
researcher

"If you're interested in the new discipline of psychedelic medicine and therapy, *Whole Medicine* is a must-read. . . . Anyone curious about psychedelic-assisted therapy should read this important manuscript."

—DARRON SMITH, PhD, PA-C, codirector at
the University of Washington Center for Novel
Therapeutics

"*Whole Medicine* is vulnerable, personal, and honors lineage. There are no promises of answers, but sincere openings for inquiries. The sacred and the secular are woven together with the acknowledgment that the natural world holds both. Readers are invited to grow alongside Rebecca in this exploration of this new phase of ancient healing. The limitations and contradictions in the field are held unbiased and appraised with a just eye. Marginalized and stigmatized voices are fully present in the reflections on what has occurred and, importantly, what is next in this psychedelic and plant medicine reemergence into the mainstream."

—COURTNEY WATSON, LMFT, founder of
Doorway Therapeutic Services and Access
to Doorways, Inc.

WHOLE MEDICINE

A GUIDE TO ETHICS
and Harm-Reduction for Psychedelic Therapy
and Plant Medicine Communities

Rebecca Martinez

with Juliette Mohr
Foreword by David Bronner

North Atlantic Books
Huichin, unceded Ohlone land
Berkeley, California

Published by
North Atlantic Books
Huichin, unceded Ohlone land
Berkeley, California

Cover art © RinaArt21 via Shutterstock
Cover design by Jess Morphew
Book design by Happenstance Type-O-Rama

Printed in Canada

Whole Medicine: A Guide to Ethics and Harm-Reduction for Psychedelic Therapy and Plant Medicine Communities is sponsored and published by North Atlantic Books, an educational nonprofit based in the unceded Ohlone land Huichin (Berkeley, CA) that collaborates with partners to develop cross-cultural perspectives; nurture holistic views of art, science, the humanities, and healing; and seed personal and global transformation by publishing work on the relationship of body, spirit, and nature.

North Atlantic Books's publications are distributed to the US trade and internationally by Penguin Random House Publisher Services. For further information, visit our website at www.northatlanticbooks.com.

DISCLAIMER: The following information is intended for general information purposes only. The publisher does not advocate illegal activities but does believe in the right of individuals to have free access to information and ideas. Any application of the material set forth in the following pages is at the reader's discretion and is their sole responsibility.

Library of Congress Cataloging-in-Publication Data

Names: Martinez, Rebecca (Founder of Alma Institute), author. | Mohr, Juliette, author. | Bronner, David, 1973- writer of foreword.
Title: Whole medicine : a guide to ethics and harm-reduction for psychedelic therapy and plant medicine communities / Rebecca Martinez with Juliette Mohr ; foreword by David Bronner.
Description: Berkeley, CA : North Atlantic Books, [2024] | Includes bibliographical references and index. | Summary: "A comprehensive framework for ethical psychedelic medicine that applies a social-justice lens to entheogenic practice and focuses on ethics, boundaries, and informed use"-- Provided by publisher.
Identifiers: LCCN 2023031748 (print) | LCCN 2023031749 (ebook) | ISBN 9781623178550 (trade paperback) | ISBN 9781623178567 (ebook)
Subjects: LCSH: Hallucinogenic drugs--Therapeutic use--Moral and ethical aspects. | Materia medica, Vegetable--Moral and ethical aspects. | Medical ethics.
Classification: LCC RM324.8 .M37 2024 (print) | LCC RM324.8 (ebook) | DDC 615.7/883--dc23/eng/20230911
LC record available at https://lccn.loc.gov/2023031748
LC ebook record available at https://lccn.loc.gov/2023031749

1 2 3 4 5 6 7 8 9 MARQUIS 28 27 26 25 24

This book includes recycled material and material from well-managed forests. North Atlantic Books is committed to the protection of our environment. We print on recycled paper whenever possible and partner with printers who strive to use environmentally responsible practices.

For Moses.

You make intergenerational healing fun.

CONTENTS

FOREWORD

I've been fortunate enough to spend the last thirty-plus years exploring consciousness for healing, growth, and celebration. Experiencing psychedelics in social and ceremonial contexts has changed the way I live and shaped my outlook on the world and my place in it. It has opened the door to profound spiritual insight and intergenerational healing, and afforded me profound, connective experiences with nature and my closest loved ones. I believe these opportunities are a human right.

Drug policy reform efforts aren't new; since the policies of prohibition and criminalization first began, there have always been those who resisted on behalf of healing plant medicines. I became passionate about these efforts in the 1990s, following a long line of activists—many of whom are now elders in the psychedelic field. For me, resistance meant advocating initially for the legalization of hemp, then medicalization of cannabis, and then ending cannabis prohibition for adult use entirely. Later, when the movements to legalize psychedelic therapies and decriminalize psychedelics gained broader momentum, I felt a clear call to throw my support and the resources of Dr. Bronner's behind these efforts, along with efforts to end the drug war completely in favor of a "treatment not jail" approach to those struggling with substance use disorders. Through Dr. Bronner's, we've been able to give millions to efforts to make psychedelics accessible to the public.

These promising modalities do not exist in a vacuum. The suffering that ails our society is complex and interwoven. This is why I see psychedelics and plant medicines fitting within a larger interdisciplinary effort to take care of our home planet, "Spaceship Earth," and all its inhabitants. For me, this has meant meaningfully supporting not only drug policy reform efforts, but also importantly, fair trade practices, labor rights, animal welfare, racial justice, climate action, and ecological stewardship. These are just a few branches of the tree of justice that we need to be tending to during these pressing times.

In the years I've been involved in this field, I've seen a surge of public enthusiasm. But while these powerful substances can catalyze deep healing and transformation in many cases, they can also amplify problematic issues like narcissism, misuse of power, and cult-like dynamics. These are issues we have to reckon with and address as we venture to safely bring psychedelics into mainstream consciousness. Fortunately, we are seeing more and more initiatives to support ethics and accountability in this field, and I believe we have further to go. We each need to look at the roles we play.

This book is a part of that effort. *Whole Medicine* is coming out at a critical time in the psychedelic field and in our collective history. With interlocking crises of our times, it has never been more urgent to anchor into our shared humanity and interrupt cycles of harm so we can move forward with more compassion and justice. This is true at a societal level, but also at a movement level. The topics in this book are expansive, yet cut to the heart of psychedelic work. Whether you are a therapist, seeker, funder, activist, or leader, you will find within these pages a rich offering of resources that can help us make the most of this global moment.

Rebecca also interviews twenty elders in this book; many are people I have come to know, love, and trust over the years. Their contributions to our collective wisdom cannot be overstated, and wise guidance should be heeded as we move through these years of rapid growth. And now with *Whole Medicine,* we are fortunate to spend time with many of them in one place.

With the first legal access program underway in Oregon, and other states soon to follow, we now have real-world opportunities to move from theory into practice at scale and show how to bring psychedelic-assisted therapy into our communities in a meaningful way. Alongside the Sheri Eckert Foundation, I see Alma Institute leading the way to ensure that equity and access are at the heart of this next period of psychedelic history. I have been struck by the integrity of their leadership, follow-through, and steadfast commitment to their core values in the face of so much urgency and pressure in the field.

In the time I have known Rebecca, I have seen her show up as a consistent, heart-centered leader and community member. She's one of the most impressive emerging leaders in the field and wise beyond her years. This book is an example of the way she leads—uplifting those around her and weaving together important truths that need to remain at the forefront of all our work. This book should become a defining text for this next era of psychedelics.

Spend time with this book: read and reread it, let it get under your skin. Grapple with the considerations in these pages. May they prompt a deeper reflection within all of us on how we got here, what healing means, and our roles in the unfolding of this historic revolution in consciousness.

With mega love and appreciation,

—David Bronner

My Background

I am a queer, cisgender, able-bodied, light-skinned Chicana. My father was born in Eagle Pass on the Texas–Mexico border, as were his mother and her parents. My grandmother speaks Spanish and "Indian" and, while she has Indigenous ancestry, the details of our family line and tribal relations were lost to assimilation. My grandfather came from Piedras Negras in Coahuila, Mexico, and he drank himself to death without ever knowing my father. Coming out of extreme poverty, my father was one of twelve children, and only half of them survived to adulthood. He left school in sixth grade to start work and help provide for the family. There is little more we know about our lineage, in my father's words, because of "fires, floods, and struggle." My mother is white and her family came out of Europe (Spain, Portugal, Ireland, England, and Germany). Her paternal grandfather came to the US from Germany as a baby, and her maternal family had immigrated to the US several generations earlier. They settled in Reno, Nevada, before making their way to Oregon.

I hold privilege due to my skin color, language, ability, education, and proximity to Eurocentric beauty standards. I was raised in a predominantly white Christian community outside of Portland, Oregon. The value and importance of cultural differences were disregarded and, while not explicitly acknowledged, whiteness was embraced as the standard. Because of this, the bicultural identity of my family was minimized and ignored for most of my upbringing.

My path to working with psychedelics has been a winding one. I was raised in a deeply religious family, the good-hearted, rebellious daughter of devout Christian parents. My first experiences with altered states of consciousness took place in the sanctuary of a Pentecostal Church. The services, marked by music, prayer, and speaking in tongues provided transcendent and often confusing experiences that I resonated with but struggled to integrate.

As I will share throughout this book, the influence of the Church on my life cannot be overstated. My parents met at a Bible study in the 1970s and I was baptized as a born-again Christian in the Columbia River (known as *Wimahl* to the Chinook people) in 1996. We were members of the Foursquare Church, an Evangelical–Pentecostal denomination focused on signs, wonders, and the coming end times. The Church is known for its music ministries and missionaries, is present in 150 countries, and has nearly seven million members worldwide.

When I was a teen, my explorations with cannabis showed me that another world could be reached by inhaling the smoke of a sticky green flower. I was enamored by the magic and weirdness I found in these places, and I sought to reconcile these experiences with the dogma of my religion. We didn't have the language for plant medicine then, but my friends and I knew that smoking the medical marijuana we'd swiped from our friends' parents' jars didn't feel like a sin; rather, it helped us feel less anxious about life and more in touch with our imaginations.

In spite of my cannabis experimentation, I remained a firm believer in the Christian faith until my late teens, when the logic of the belief system started to unravel. When I graduated from high school at age seventeen, I dove into religion by attending Bible college, mainly to alleviate my creeping doubts. However, my exposure to people who held other worldviews, as well as my acceptance of my own queerness and the realization that I did not believe in hell as a literal place, resulted in an increasingly shaky commitment to the religion by the time I graduated. Grappling with my doubts and internal shifts was complicated because I had led the music ministry for several churches for years, and thus held a high level of visibility.

Several traumatic events happened in my family during the years I was married and gave birth to my son. They involved cancer diagnoses, a police shooting, and the incarceration of two immediate family members. What was left of my spiritual life dissolved, eroded by the realities around me, and in its absence, I embraced an icy atheism that sheltered me for several years. For me, God was dead.

Meeting the Medicines

The mushrooms found me a few years later when I began to come out the other side. I was newly divorced and living with my small son in an urban farm community with several other families. A fellow mother in the house, an herbalist, was being trained to work with psilocybin mushrooms and offered to hold a session with me. I agreed. While I had consumed a lot of cannabis during my teens, I had never had an experience with psychedelics. I felt curious and open to the wisdom they might hold.

A few weeks later, I was sitting on the floor of our ornate treehouse in a big-leaf maple tree, drinking hot earthy water and chewing the softened *Psilocybe cyanescens* mushrooms at the bottom of my cup. This August afternoon was a pivotal day in my life, as significant as the birth of my son, the day of my divorce, and the night my father was shot by police during a mental health crisis when I was eight months pregnant. These humble mushrooms enabled me to encounter buried memories and wounds I'd tried to forget and helped me contend with my grief and loss of faith. I was visited by ancestors on both sides. I began to soften my armor and become tender enough to feel again. And for the first time in several years, I could sense the warm presence of something holy. Only this time, there was no separation between myself and this entity; it was a sacred communion I'd been craving throughout my young life. It felt like being drawn into the arms of God, and hearing the words, "Welcome back. I'm not who you thought I was."

I experienced communion with spirit that I thought had been lost for good. As I integrated the experience in the coming days and weeks, I was astounded by the way this daylong journey of the soul helped me relate to my life with more compassion, trust, and agility. My tolerance for mystery increased and so did my ability to forgive. My impulse to control my behavior, my circumstances, and the people around me began to subside.

Eight years of psychedelic healing followed, marked by experimentation, trial, and error, as I discovered the powers of these stigmatized substances. My loved ones (many of them seasoned psychonauts) and I continued to explore expanded states with a variety of settings and substances. I found that each experience had its own teachings, regardless of whether we had stayed up all night dancing to live music or silently traversed the depths of our souls beside a babbling brook. The freedom to experiment this way is a privilege few are afforded. I came to revere these experiences as sacred. I learned that healing doesn't just look like nitty-gritty processing and hard work. It is treading on new paths through play, celebration, pleasure, mystery, and relationships.

Entering the Field

I began to "hold space" for friends as they embarked on their own adventures of consciousness. *Holding space* is a term that has become commonplace in the field. It means "to be fully present with someone" and "to foster an environment suited for vulnerable states." My first experiences holding space were in a harm-reduction capacity as a trip-sitter, often in less-than-ideal scenarios, where I was the only (or most) sober person present. A trip-sitter refers to a designated person responsible for the safety and well-being of people consuming mind-altering substances. Their responsibility is not to guide the experience, but to help manage risks and provide a safe, supportive presence.

Soon, I was being asked to trip-sit for friends and acquaintances on more intentional mushroom sessions. I discovered the hard way that mentorship and consultation are essential for people who find themselves in support roles. These early experiences taught me a great deal about how to hold space for people, and the feedback I received was as humbling as it was encouraging. It turns out, good intentions are not enough. We need ongoing inner-work and practical tools in order to meaningfully support the people who come to us in search of expansive experiences.

I was at a Paul Stamets talk in Portland, Oregon, in 2018 when I first heard of Oregon's effort to create legal access to adult-use psilocybin. A year later, I found myself on staff at the Measure 109 campaign, training volunteers around the state and hitting the streets to gather thousands of ballot signatures. The effort was successful. The bill passed in November 2020, and suddenly my home state became a testing ground for therapeutic access to psilocybin and the focus of national attention.

I was concerned the program would be costly and hard to access, so I became deeply involved in the state's subsequent rulemaking process. I cofounded a grass-roots education and advocacy group. From there, I was recruited to numerous local and national working groups and committees that were seeking meaning-ful ways to create equitable access to these potentially life-altering substances. I wished to help build the safest, soundest, most compassionate, and transforma-tional social system possible for mushroom use.

In 2021, I founded Alma Institute, a nonprofit training program for psilocy-bin facilitators in Oregon. I work alongside a diverse, trusted group of colleagues who hold decades of combined experience with entheogens, psychedelic ther-apy, and trauma-informed care, as well as licenses in mental health and natural medicine. We have set out to help steward the mainstreaming of psychedelics with integrity. Alma Institute became licensed as a private career school and our curriculum was approved by the Oregon Health Authority, enabling us to certify facilitators for licensure under the Psilocybin Services Act. Our mission is to strengthen and diversify the field of psychedelic healing. My work centers on creating models for community use of psychedelics that are safe, ethical, and culturally attuned. It is an honor to have been welcomed into the psychedelic field and to be able to share my perspectives in this book alongside so many of the people I deeply admire.

My Orientation and Lineage of Practice

This life is far too mysterious for us to be matter-of-fact about everything, and after two decades of participation in a fundamentalist religious institution, I'm resistant to any belief system that professes to know "the way it is." In my view, spirituality is best expressed as love in action. Beyond that, I don't have many answers to offer, and this book will rarely point to absolutes. What I can offer is sincere inquiry and a reflection on recurring themes that show up in fractals and merit our attention. I believe our bodies are where we bridge the secular and the sacred and discover they are not separate.

I have found certain frameworks and practices that resonate deeply with my experience of the world and guide my movement through it. Much of my (un) learning has to do with how we become more present and how we create space for more justice and pleasure. Here are some of the systems of practice I am committed to and/or have trained in:

Healing Justice (via Cara Page and the Kindred Southern Healing Justice Collective): a framework that aims to address widespread generational trauma from systemic violence and oppression by reviving ancestral healing practices and building new, more inclusive ones.

Somatic Abolitionism (via Resmaa Menakem): an individual and communal effort to free our bodies—and the US—from their long enslavement to white body supremacy and racialized trauma.

Transformative Justice: a political framework and approach for responding to violence, harm, and abuse. At its most basic, it seeks to respond to violence without creating more violence. This framework seeks to transform the root causes of harm.

Emergent Strategy (via adrienne maree brown): a strategy for building complex patterns and systems of change through relatively small interactions" and "an adaptive, relational way of being."[1]

Harm-Reduction: a risk management approach focused on kindness, compassion, and respect for people who use psychoactive substances. This field of practice emerged from groups of people who have been criminalized—drug users and sex workers—and people who support them.

Permaculture: an approach to land management and design that adopts arrangements observed in flourishing natural ecosystems. This set of design principles is rooted in whole systems thinking, and is intrinsic to many Indigenous land-tending practices.

In addition to the above disciplines, my cosmology has been shaped by the teachings of Indigenous cultures around the world that hold there is no separation between humans and nature. Many of the themes in this book draw on Indigenous wisdom that is held and lived out within traditional communities, and it is my intent to recognize and be in reciprocity with them wherever possible.

My conceptualization of healing and justice work is shaped by the work and examples of adrienne maree brown, Robin Wall Kimmerer, Leah Penniman, Prentis Hemphill, Kai Cheng Thom, Resmaa Menakem, Esteban Kelly, Gloria Anzaldúa, Tricia Hersey, and many others. At the intersection of psychedelics and social justice, I look to Diana Quinn, Claudia Cuentas, Hanifa Nayo Washington, Ismail Ali, and many heart-aligned medicine keepers and elders who cannot be named due to the risks and impacts of prohibition and criminalization.

I am also the product of many people who have poured into me over the years: pastors, educators, spiritual teachers, social justice leaders, neighbors, healers, ancestors, elders, mentors, advisors, the brilliant humans who contributed to this book, and my team at Alma Institute. The ideas I'll put forth in this book cannot be separated from this web of relationships and knowledge sharing that has produced me.

About Our Guests

This book features numerous guests and interviews in various formats. These guests are esteemed colleagues, mentors, and leaders in the space who have helped shape my understanding of the Essential Elements of Practice. Many of them are also dear friends and people I share a community with. Their subject matter expertise and professional experience help fill in my knowledge gaps and provide a more comprehensive look at the topics we'll be exploring. I hope this collaborative approach enriches your experience and demonstrates that power sharing is a worthwhile endeavor. Together, we know a lot.

The conversations explore complex topics and are often open-ended by design. I hope that after reading, you will take the time to get familiar with these individuals and support their work, rich projects, and bodies of knowledge that embody and inform the concepts introduced here.

Limitations

When I was asked to write this book, I almost said no. It felt nearly impossible to contribute something wholly good to a space where it feels like there are risks on all sides. I am painfully aware of my own limitations in experience and understanding.

I realized the only way I could offer this book in good integrity would be to do my best to model the principles put forth within its pages: that is, to involve community, share power, and do the inner-work of being aware of my own shadows and shortcomings. I have been fortunate to interview and involve some of the people who have guided me and who hold important voices in this field.

I am also sitting with my own fears:

I may overlook important truths.

I may contradict myself.

I may offend people or make them uncomfortable.

I may unintentionally hurt the very groups I wish to uplift and support.

I may be misunderstood or have my words taken out of context.

I may go too far or not far enough.

I may not do justice to the topics we cover.

People may reject the ideas put forth or those who offer them.

I will certainly not be perfect.

It is inevitable that many of the above fears, and other surprises, will happen along the way. I welcome feedback and disagreement; we will certainly not agree on everything contained within these pages, and that is part of being in community together. I aspire to hold onto ideas loosely, with a willingness to evolve. My hope is that this book further catalyzes community discourse and fuels the good work already being done in this field. My hope is that we can learn from one another as we fumble through the coming years.

Thank you for coming on this journey with me. Here we go.

INTRODUCTION

The Moment

It's no secret that psychedelics are coming back on the scene. What may have seemed like a fringe movement, limited to psychedelic enthusiasts and optimistic researchers, has now become a diverse global push for drug policy reform and a call to reexamine mainstream cultural beliefs around psychedelics. In light of a growing body of research, substances like psilocybin, MDMA, and LSD are gaining attention for their potential to help treat many ailments. At the top of this list are depression, anxiety, PTSD, substance-use disorders, and end-of-life distress.

Running parallel to this research is a growing community of people who believe it is a human right to experiment with one's consciousness. Many among them have set out on healing journeys with earth-based medicines such as mushrooms, cannabis, ayahuasca, iboga, and mescaline-containing cacti. Recent widespread awakenings around systemic injustice have called into question the prohibition and criminalization of substances and the people who use them. These forces have coalesced into the current surge of interest in psychedelics and a wave of new legislation.

Like all decentralized movements, there is a rich diversity of approaches, agendas, and belief systems housed under what is being called a "psychedelic resurgence." Like a mushroom fruiting from the forest floor, we are witnessing a phenomenon that is shifting by the moment, transforming so rapidly that we can see it change before our eyes. It's a field of practice that stands to disrupt entire industries and, some have claimed, revolutionize not only mental healthcare, but human consciousness.

Amidst this surge of public interest from seekers, onlookers, would-be healers, and profiteers, important questions are coming to the forefront. Should the agents of expanded consciousness be owned and patented? What does it mean to be in right relationship? What can we learn from, and how can we honor, humanity's legacy of practice with entheogens—a legacy that began with Indigenous communities well before the launch of Nixon's drug war or the first waves of Western institutional research? How do practices of consumption that are considered recreational—such as play, experimentation, and celebration—fit into a public conversation heavily focused on psychedelics as a therapeutic tool?

At first glance, it may seem like this surge came out of nowhere. As we look closer, we find that there is a global legacy of practice that never stopped during the time of prohibition. Within Indigenous communities in North, Central, and South America, and secret circles in major cities around the United States and beyond, people have never stopped gathering in groups to experience altered states of consciousness. While this underground movement has held important wisdom and helped many people along their paths, it has also exposed vulnerabilities that we now have to contend with as prohibition begins to crumble and the mainstream public becomes more open to the potential benefits of psychedelics.

The Need

Stories that detail a spectrum of ethical violations and abuses ranging from disappointing to profoundly disturbing have been surfacing for years. It's no longer possible to write these off as isolated incidents or the behavior of a few. What's becoming clear is that the matrix of factors involved with expanded states of consciousness exposes both participants and those who hold space to unique risks. These amplified dynamics make even the best-intentioned people vulnerable to oversights, errors, and lapses in judgment. While the potential for benefit and healing is great, so is the potential for deep harm and retraumatization to ourselves and those seeking help. We are playing with a fire that is set to spread across the globe. Will it be a fire that warms or one that destroys?

Those of us who have experienced the transformative potential of psychedelics are tasked with helping steward their shift into the mainstream, whether we consented to this duty or not. Some of us have been practicing for decades, and some are newcomers. To a disconnected culture, we may all be seen as experts and leaders in the coming years. So, what is our responsibility in this great unfolding? What messages do we wish to send the world about these powerful and misunderstood substances? How can we embrace their potential from a grounded perspective, one marked with self-awareness and balance, rooted in heart, nuance, and integrity?

This book explores Essential Elements of Psychedelic Practice. Whether you are a curious seeker or a seasoned practitioner, this book aims to edify you on your path and provide guideposts so you know what questions to ask and flags to spot on your journey. For those who provide support, whether grassroots guides, casual trip-sitters, or psychedelic therapists, this book offers important considerations to help you shape and strengthen your practice.

For all of us, this book seeks to serve as an immunological offering to the psychedelic field. Spending time with the uncomfortable and shadowy parts of ourselves and our communities early on can help us prevent catastrophic harm later. One of my mentors says, "Little deaths help prevent big deaths." May this simple offering help us find and address problems, heal wounds, and nourish our personal and communal practices. In doing so, perhaps this psychedelic resurgence can become a deeply grounded, positive social movement with the integrity to last.

About This Book

I am writing this book not as a therapist or a self-proclaimed healer; I am writing as a community member who has sat on both sides of the altar. I earned a degree in Spiritual Leadership from a small Bible college and later went to school for massage therapy, which provided me with a foundational understanding of the therapeutic relationship. While I have served in a leadership and support role for people experiencing mind-altering substances since 2016, I am also an avid explorer of my own consciousness, a sexual assault survivor, and a former staff member of an Evangelical megachurch who lived through years of spiritual abuse and manipulation.

I am setting out to offer advocacy for clients and resources for facilitators. Along the way, you may notice nature-based allusions and metaphors. I am trained in a systems thinking perspective rooted in regenerative ecosystem study that examines how parts are interconnected and the macro–micro interplay between individual and collective experience.

Because I have witnessed firsthand what can happen in circumstances with major power differentials, I have concerns about the risks of training a generation of self-proclaimed gurus or propping up dogmatic communities where groupthink reigns supreme. Instead, I am interested in exploring what happens when we close the power gaps between client and facilitator, trip-sitter, and journeyer. I am interested in reducing the discrepancies of knowledge that make abuse possible by educating seekers on what they can and should expect. I am interested in doing what we can to prevent harm and offering practical tools for accountability and repair.

Ultimately, my hope is that we can find ways to engage these ancient sacraments not only to heal and enrich our individual lives, but also to collectively establish right relationship with these substances and their origins. Through this, I believe we will find that their teachings can help humanity navigate these unprecedented times with more grace, hope, and justice.

This book is written with the aim of distilling the core themes that must be grappled with when encountering psychedelics. It highlights thirteen core themes, which I call the Essential Elements of Practice. These include: Inner-Work, Presence, Shadow, Discernment, Community, Power, Pacing, Harm-Reduction, Consent, Accountability, History, Reciprocity, and Hope.

Each of these Elements of Practice has relevance for psychedelic work, and like a fractal, when multiplied to a global context, has major implications for our society at large. Over time and with scale, healthy expressions of these elements within ourselves and our medicine communities have the power to shape society. This is why spending time with these Elements of Practice can be so impactful—if each of us is a drop, we collectively make up a river of transformative healing potential.

This book is written with intentional use in mind; thus, it does not seek to cover the more extreme aspects of what can occur in festival environments, cases of accidental consumption, encountering people mid-crisis, or cases where people have consumed unknown or combinations of substances. Resources such as *The Manual of Psychedelic Support* and X. Razma's *Guide for Guides* provide in-depth, practical education around trip-sitting and harm-reduction within these less controlled contexts.

Who This Is For

This book is written for *psychedelic space holders* (a catchall term including psychedelic therapists, facilitators, guides, and trip-sitters) as well as the *psychedelic curious*. It is intended to help establish a shared language and spark conversations within our practices, medicine circles, organizations, and personal lives.

The mainstreaming of psychedelics will not take one singular shape. In fact, the contexts in which one can consume consciousness-altering substances vary widely and will continue to broaden. That said, these contexts can be grouped into a few main groups with key differences.

Therapeutic: Psychedelic-assisted therapies are set to become a history-making disruptive industry that advocates say could revolutionize mental health as we know it. This model entails the intentional use of psychedelics with the express intention of addressing an ailment, most often a mental health challenge, involving the mind, body, heart, and soul. Psychedelic therapy is usually conducted by trained mental health professionals or underground practitioners who use psychedelic substances as an adjunct to therapeutic modalities. This model has recently been popularized by groups such as the MAPS protocol for MDMA-assisted therapy; and a variety of groups—such as Usona Institute and Johns Hopkins Center for Psychedelic & Consciousness Research—that have designed protocols for the therapeutic use of psilocybin, DMT, and many other promising compounds, in addition to the many decades of underground citizen science that paved the way for these institutions.

Ceremonial: Anchored in sacred Indigenous practices, the ceremonial use of plant medicines and sacred brews goes back millennia. From the traditional use of yagé, or ayahuasca, by tribes throughout the Amazon basin, to sacred mushroom ceremonies or *veladas,* in what is now called Oaxaca,

Mexico, working with psychoactive plants is a quintessentially human act. These ceremonies exist within a biocultural context, and the rituals, songs, and practices that take place within traditional ceremonial settings cannot be separated from the people, land, history, language, and cosmology of those who developed the practices. These ceremonies were and are still conducted at key moments of the year or during the participants' life cycle for prayer, healing, rites of passage, and communion with the divine.

Peer Support/Recreational: Environments in which the consumption of psychedelics has been destigmatized and normalized. This often takes place in friend groups, group gatherings, or festival environments. Ideally, shared agreements are centered and all participants are on the same page regarding intentions, expectations, and safety plans. The psychedelic field has begun to acknowledge that nonmedical and celebratory use is valid; it can also be healing in its own right.

Solo Journeying: The use of psychedelic substances, drugs, brews, or plant allies for healing, insight, and personal growth. Many people, especially more experienced journeyers, may choose to engage with psychedelics alone in the privacy of their homes, out in nature, or in retreat settings.

This book will not provide simple, easy-to-replicate steps to healing with psychedelics, or an easy formula for being an ethical facilitator. To claim this would be not only arrogant but impossible. What I will provide are key considerations and an exploration of the potential downstream impacts of various ways of working. I am asking you to do the work of applying these core themes and principles to your specific context.

Some Foundational Principles

We can't assume we all have the same orientation simply due to our shared interest in psychedelics. I see the value of discourse, disagreement, and diversity of thought. I also acknowledge that I have blind spots, incomplete ideas, and contradictions. With further learning, I might find things written in this book that I'm unable to stand by in the future. Still, I am writing this book upon a few key beliefs:

1. Life is mysterious, complex, and irrefutably sacred. Humans don't and can't have all the answers.

2. Being alive is the work of reconciling our physical and mystical experiences.

3. We all have trauma; like most things, it exists on a spectrum rather than a binary.

4. Psychedelics do more than alter our perception; they allow us to journey into real planes of existence beyond physical realms.

5. There is an inherent spiritual aspect to life on earth and, as such, working with psychedelics entails engaging with spirituality.

6. At the core of our healing work are issues of power, consent, autonomy, and belonging.

7. We all hold an innate healing intelligence and the capacity to heal.

8. Individual healing is an illusion. Healing happens in an interconnected web.

9. Until we learn to explore our shadows, practice accountability, and hold space for many truths at once, we will stay caught in a cycle of harm and othering.

10. Taking psychedelics isn't going to magically fix the world. We need radical systems changes for that.

11. The above two activities are not mutually exclusive.

What Is Whole Medicine?

The topic of healing is a huge one. It's a question that is central to our existence as conscious beings who experience pain and connection. When we reflect deeply on the notion of healing, there is a common thread that emerges—the idea of repair, restoration, and accessing our innate wholeness. The notion of medicine can conjure many associations, from pharmaceuticals to memories of soul-stirring experiences. What connects these concepts is the potential to help us: body, mind, and soul. To do us *good*—usually on a personal level.

Whole medicine proposes that healing is, in its very essence, collective. It denies the fantasy that some of us can heal while looking the other way at the harms being done around us. It calls us to begin within ourselves, become aware of the conditions we are steeped in, and show up in service of change.

Whole medicine is not just about feeling better; it is about living differently. Whole medicine insists that we do not stop with our own healing, but that we allow ourselves to be interrupted by the worthy pursuit of a more just and beautiful world. Whole medicine acknowledges that when we really let the medicines in . . . they could change everything by changing us.

For the transformative potential of psychedelics to be realized, we must extend beyond tending to the imbalances and pain in our own lives. It will require that we confront our collective shadows in order to disrupt the upstream legacies of violence and domination we have collectively inherited. We must expand our field of vision to see how we are situated within our family systems, local communities, ecosystems, and the world. We must imagine what is possible when we liberate ourselves from these cycles and return to the relational communion that is the heart of life as conscious beings.

These principles are obvious to many intact Indigenous communities around the world. Healing work means remembering and reconnecting with these truths. In order for medicine to be whole, it needs to be reconnected with its multitude of expressions that exist beyond the echo chambers of psychedelia and woven in meaningful ways back into the world around us. Imagine what could happen when carefully stewarded ancestral practices consciously intersect with the cultural forces of sacred activism, land tending, food justice, the arts, community, family, culture, love.

This isn't a question of how psychedelics can be heroes that make the world better. It's about stepping outside of our sense of heroism to see the healing forces that exist all around us, and discovering generative collaboration and partnership across modalities. It's an inquiry into how we can weave our default realities and our travels through expanded states. It points to the fractal relationship between the individual and the collective. That edge is where the magic and wonder happen. How do we go about this weaving of worlds? We'll have to figure out this unfolding together.

About the Language Used in This Book

In the psychedelic field, sometimes it seems like we need a dictionary to keep all the terms we use straight. Here are some details about the language used within these pages.

PSYCHEDELICS: I use *psychedelics* as a catchall term to include psychoactive compounds that are naturally occurring and synthesized. These include the "classical psychedelics" such as LSD, psilocybin, DMT, and mescaline (and their various sources) as well as the broader family of substances including MDMA, ketamine, and a growing list of others.

PSYCHEDELIC HEALING: I use this term interchangeably with *psychedelic work, medicine work, journey work, ceremony,* and *psychedelic experience.* The practice of consuming a psychedelic for the purpose of growth, insight, and/or healing.

ENTHEOGEN: This usually refers to a psychoactive plant or fungi used ceremonially by traditional communities. These include psilocybin, ayahuasca, peyote, iboga, and others. Also commonly referred to as *plant medicine* (though this term has wide-ranging definitions) and *sacred earth medicine.*

DRUGS: I use this term to refer to mind-altering substances, specifically those that have been criminalized through the Controlled Substances Act. In these chapters, I attempt to be specific whether I am talking about all substances or psychedelics.

SACRAMENT: A substance used in intentional or ceremonial contexts; could be naturally occurring or synthetic.

FACILITATOR: A person responsible for the safety and well-being of someone consuming psychedelics. Also referred to as a guide or trip-sitter.

PSYCHEDELIC THERAPIST: A mental health professional trained in psychedelic-assisted therapy (PAT), the use of psychedelics to treat or address various mental health concerns.

JOURNEYER: The person having the psychedelic experience. Used interchangeably with *client, practitioner,* and *seeker.*

INTEGRATION: The process of making meaning out of the insights gained in a psychedelic experience.

NOSC: A nonordinary state of consciousness. I use this term interchangeably with *altered states* and *expanded states.* The state someone experiences while under the influence of a psychoactive substance (can also be initiated through other means).

There may be other terms used throughout the book that are unfamiliar to you. Where possible, I will provide a definition. If you are unsure what a term means, it is worth taking the time to look it up. For terms with various meanings, please use the content of this book to provide additional context and clarification.

CHAPTER 1

Inner-Work

Inner-work has held a convoluted meaning throughout my life. Realizing the ways the idea had been co-opted was an integral step in my own path to healing. During my time in Bible college, I felt I was forever standing at a crossroads where I had to choose between my own experience and sense of inner ethics, and the rules of the Church; the two were often in conflict.

For example, as a leader in the music ministry, I was once required to play "God Bless America" during a large weekend church service; when I protested, I was told that if I refused, I would be placed on sabbatical. On a tour through Israel, I listened to our guide say unrepeatable things about the people of Palestine, and when I brought it up to a leader, I was urged not to "rock the boat." I witnessed a close mentor express homophobic ideas, while I was quietly aware of and concealing my own queerness.

I began to notice that I had been hiding behind my belief system, even as my doubts grew, to avoid taking actual accountability for my life. The metrics for assessing one's personal practice weren't based on the impacts we had in the world around us or whether we were moving toward our personal goals; they depended on how closely we aligned with the institution of the Church. Within this system, I always had something outside of myself that I could point to as justification for my behavior (even if it was problematic or harmful), or an easy-out of repenting for my sins and moving forward with a "clean slate." This is why it was so freeing and terrifying when I finally left the faith at twenty-two. I no longer had to contort my ideals to fit the Church, but I also had no convenient escape route if things went sideways. I had to start being responsible for my life.

In this way, I believe my true inner-work began as I left the Church and started to peel back the layers of conditioning that had shaped my personality. I believe inner-work is not just about addressing our personal shortcomings so we can heal or be happy; it is also about identifying and shedding whatever keeps us from aligning with ethics that support life. It is about identifying where we have been harmed, but also where we are the ones doing harm. On one hand, I had to let go of the self-loathing and sense of inadequacy that was enabled by the Church. I had to look at my own internalized homophobia and other harmful beliefs. I began to unpack the extreme perfectionism, self-doubt, and fear of failure that had been driving my

decisions. I deconstructed an embedded self-righteousness and became a more curi-
ous and accepting person. I quieted the fear of theistic surveillance and realized that
not everything was so serious.

For me, working with psychedelics feels starkly different from religion. They don't
come with a prescribed belief system to measure my insights against. They rarely tell
me what to do; they open me to a deeper soulful level of being that responds to each
question with another question. The medicines are so much more compassionate
with me than I was prepared for. They hold a mirror up to me and, instead of berat-
ing me for my shortcomings, they say things like, "What if you aren't really broken?"
and "You've been carrying a lot more than you need to," and "Hey, stop your fretting
and look at that cool dragonfly."

As grueling as inner-work can be, it can also be deeply relieving and rewarding.
And . . . it will catch up to us eventually, so we might as well lean in.

Defining Inner-Work

I define inner-work as the practice of self-reflection and inquiry to better understand your beliefs, traumas, actions, reactions, and biases. This active practice
is the basis for any sustainable growth, healing, and change. Inner-work does
not have a defined end date; it is an ongoing practice that we commit to for life.

We begin here with inner-work, because one major site of psychedelic healing is our own consciousness. Psychedelics act on our awareness, perspectives,
and understanding of the world. But they do not do so in a vacuum: they interact
with our existing preconceptions, our inner worlds. The benefits, limitations,
and dangers of psychedelics are shaped by our capacity to prepare for, experience, and integrate openings in our consciousness. The inner world is one we
need to be familiar with in order to safely traverse it.

Our relationships to ourselves and the world are shaped by lived experience. When we experience harm, natural survival mechanisms activate to protect us from feeling that pain again. While these adaptations help keep us safe
in the short term, they can also armor us so heavily that we struggle to connect
with those around us, or cloud our sense of self and leave us feeling lost. Inner-
work enables us to recognize adaptations that no longer benefit us and to chart
a path toward the conditions we need to heal and thrive. There are of course
some things that cannot be undone. In addition to our own pain, the field of
epigenetics demonstrates what original cultures have long known: that we also
carry a profound inheritance from the generations before us.

For those who seek healing, inner-work is the heart of the journey. It requires
that we quiet the noise of the world and make space for the messages living in

our hearts, minds, bodies, and spirits. It asks us to get curious so we can get reacquainted with ourselves and gain self-compassion and awareness. From this place, we can actively choose how to engage with ourselves, others, and the world—a choice that happens continuously—rather than reactively fumbling through life. *Without time spent "doing the work," we risk continuing harmful cycles we are not even aware are playing out as we engage with psychedelics.* We risk living our whole lives without bringing into consciousness the roots and tendrils of our wounds, and how those tendrils affect others. We risk, too, withholding the gifts and dreams that lie buried beneath these wounds, denying our greatest inheritance.

Inner-work is about self-responsibility and accountability, but most of all, it is an act of radical hope and love.

Exploring Inner-Work

Spending time on inner-work is a nonnegotiable starting point for anyone who wants to partake in, serve, or steward medicine responsibly. This is particularly important for those in leadership and field-building positions (e.g., training program leaders and trainers, scientists, investors/donors, policymakers, journalists). Generally, inner-work helps us shift away from a reactionary stance to a more intentional and accountable one. It helps us feel more connected to ourselves and find more spaciousness and choice, and as a result, make fewer excuses for ourselves.

WHY ARE WE HERE?

Everything that unfolds in psychedelics next—personally, interpersonally, and in the field at large—will be a result of what's happening right now in the hearts, bodies, minds, and spirits of those who are participating as stewards. This is a sobering thought given that all of us are also navigating a time of tremendous change, disruption, and yes, collective trauma. It is impossible to separate our inner worlds from the actions we take and the worlds we build.

Beginning with the quiet. Beginning with a pause.

As you read this chapter, and all that follow, I encourage you to take regular breaks to check in with your breath. With compassion, slow down and notice what's coming up for you. There may be some surprises.

To start, I invite you to reflect: why are *you* here?

Perhaps you've arrived at an exploration of consciousness out of curiosity. Many people find their way to psychedelics through a friend or family member who has had a direct important or transformative experience. Maybe you read a book or saw a documentary that challenged your preconceptions about substance use.

Mental health challenges—so widespread in our time—might have led you down a seeker's path, opening a willingness to try anything that might offer some relief. The need for new options helps reduce the once-powerful stigma, and the growing body of research instills confidence. There are growing numbers of therapists, mental health professionals, and others who—confronted daily with the failings of the prevailing biomedical model—are desperate for psychedelics to help us address the root cause of all that ails us. We are now seeing policy initiatives around the United States with unlikely spokespeople such as doctors, military veterans, and hospice workers driving the conversation.

Still, others have been on a personal path of exploration in relationship with sacred plants and psychoactive substances for many years. Perhaps you work in therapeutic contexts (grassroots and aboveground) supporting people on their journeys or partake independently as an expression of cognitive liberty.

Inner-work is the place we will return to again and again, no matter how many journeys we take or people we support. There will never be a time when inner-work isn't essential to staying in right relationship and preventing harm within ourselves, our relationships, and the psychedelic field at large.

WHERE WE'VE BEEN

As we embark on an exploration of inner-work, it is important to remember that many of us were taught to view mind-altering substances with fear and suspicion, believing they would scramble our brains or prompt us to leap out a window. This tale is one shaped by the drug war, and the West's hyper-rationalist fear of the mystical (or just the unknown). As a result, many of us disregard experiences that deviate from this norm as fantasies or hallucinations. This difficulty or inability to see other perspectives is a huge contributor to our social ills, and one we must actively work against as we seek to build a healthy psychedelic field.

In spite of this centuries-old fear and the forces of prohibition and criminalization, there is a diverse web of deeply rooted mystical practice that was never forgotten. It was sheltered and revived thanks to the courage of traditional lineage keepers, grassroots community practitioners, activists, and people for whom cognitive liberty and spiritual practice were more important than the risks of breaking the law.

The exploration of expanded states is an ancient human phenomenon. In Indigenous traditions around the globe, the holiest days of the year and important rites of passage are often marked with practices that transported human minds into other states of being. Consider the peyote ceremonies of the Indigenous people of Turtle Island, the meditation rituals of Eastern Buddhist traditions, the drumming and dance of African tribal communities, or the vision quests of the First Nations people of Australia. Fasting, drumming, dancing, chanting, breathwork, and consumption of psychoactive plants and brews have all been used to facilitate the shifts in consciousness that, some could argue, are part of what make us human. Perhaps there is something innate within us that yearns for the illumination of our lives.

UNPACKING OUR PARADIGMS

With self-inquiry, we can begin to identify the underlying beliefs we hold to be true about the world, society, and ourselves. As we orient ourselves to psychedelics, which are reality-bending creatures unto themselves, we need to first ground into a clear-eyed understanding of our starting points. This is essential for a couple of reasons.

Our beliefs—whether conscious or not—are the source of our actions. We often believe our default worldviews are both universal and neutral. For example, as young children, our sense of reality is shaped by our lived experiences and what we're taught by our caregivers. As we grow older and learn more about the world, we discover there are myriad ways to live. Along the path of maturing, many of us will have the epiphany that, in fact, *my experience is not everyone's experience.* Taken further, we can discover that *my truth is not your truth, and my healing path may be different from your healing path. My thriving may not be the same as your thriving.* Moving beyond one's own sense of universality is a humbling and ongoing practice.

When we believe our way is *right,* this implies that other ways are *wrong,* and creates an internal hierarchy in which we are more correct, righteous, whole, or important than the people around us or those in other communities. When this happens, we run the risk of projecting this onto the world around us. If we succumb to a sense of superiority, we lose the ability to hear one another, lead with integrity, and support people whose lived experience differs from our own. Taken to an extreme, this sense of rightness can manifest as authoritarianism and a desire to control or extinguish those who exist in opposition to our beliefs.

What does this have to do with psychedelics? A lot. Our lived experiences, beliefs, and attitudes follow us wherever we go. The more self-awareness we can cultivate, the clearer we will be and the more responsibility we can take on when we (even unintentionally) try to impose our beliefs, priorities, or needs onto someone else. These dynamics are amplified when we hold positions of social power by being a member of a dominant group in a given society. Dominant groups vary around the world. In the United States, this social power generally comes with being white, cisgender, straight, able-bodied, English-speaking, educated, and having access to wealth and/or economic mobility.

Not appreciating the subjectivity of experience can lead to inflicting significant harm on others, especially those in marginalized communities. Subtle forms of racism, transphobia, ableism, elitism, and xenophobia are all around us daily—personally, interpersonally, and systemically. Rather than being just about individual conscious actions, we need to recognize that these forms of oppression live among us as part of the dominant culture. Without us doing the inner-work to proactively acknowledge their reality and presence, they can and do creep into the psychedelic space—our organizations, societies, and social circles.

The first step in preventing this is recognizing that we each have subjective beliefs. They may be closely held and well supported, but they will always be a product of one's own lived experience and inquiry. It's incredible what this acknowledgment can do for our personal relationships and sense of belonging in the world. Suddenly, we don't have to be correct in order to belong. We don't have to change anyone's mind. There is space in the circle of community for my experience and others that contradict mine. From the skeptical critic to the hopeful seeker, one thing binds us: we recognize that psychedelics hold power and carry cultural significance during this historic moment. We do not have to exist in a circle of homogeneity; in fact, it's essential to our health as a society that we don't.

Inner-Work in the Medicine Space

The following is an inexhaustive list of traits that can be seen in people who are engaged in their inner-work. These are traits that in my experience reflect psychologically safe, healthy individuals. They are essential qualities to cultivate to fully realize the benefits of psychedelics, and to look for in a psychedelic facilitator.

1. They hold self-knowledge. They can identify why they are the way they are, without attaching to those traits as permanent or excusable.

2. They are in touch with clear, prosocial ideals, values, and ethics.

3. They are working to create coherence between their ideals and actions; they act in alignment with their stated values.

4. They are aware of their weaknesses, can speak openly about them without defensiveness or fragility.

5. They apologize and make meaningful changes when needed. They avoid making excuses for themselves.

6. They "own their part." In a conflict, they take responsibility and can identify how their actions, reactions, or beliefs contributed.

7. They receive feedback with willingness to reflect and offer feedback from a place of compassion.

8. They view growth and healing as lifelong processes and recognize that perfectionism is at odds with meaningful inner-work.

9. They embrace setbacks from a place of accountability and self-compassion.

10. They hold curiosity about their shadow sides and are working to understand and transform them. They can answer the question, "What are you working on healing or shifting in yourself right now?"

REASONS WE AVOID INNER-WORK

It is uncomfortable. Accepting feedback or looking at parts of ourselves that we're not proud of often triggers feelings of guilt, anger, blame, and shame. These can be associated with feelings of rejection that impact our ability to feel safe in the world. Inner-work is inherently challenging, and the process is lifelong. *In a culture that has taught us to run from discomfort, inner-work demands endless self-compassion as well as accountability.*

We're in denial. In an effort to avoid difficult emotions, we may resort to toxic positivity, defensiveness, and refusal to accept feedback. In extreme cases, this can manifest as narcissistic tendencies, which we'll discuss later on. In spite of the fear of rejection, confronting our weaknesses or less flattering traits can actually help us access *more* safety. Along with belonging to a community, self-reflection can lead to action toward positive change and more prosocial behaviors.

It is vulnerable. We have been taught to avoid vulnerability and associate it with weakness. Ironically, inner-work can give us more power through building awareness and understanding. This increases our agency to make decisions we can stand behind and the courage to course-correct when we fall short of our ideals or standards.

We don't know how. Modern culture doesn't value or promote self-reflection. It promotes winning and advancement. These pursuits avoid reflection by focusing one's attention externally and rewarding efforts to dominate the "other."

We may also be in an environment or surrounded by people who don't challenge us to grow. Maintenance of a status quo—even when it is dysfunctional—can sometimes be prioritized within the family system, organizational culture, religious system, or social groups. This can create added difficulty for those who want to grow and evolve, as it can mean breaking ranks with loved ones or social norms.

FOR JOURNEYERS

Below are a few considerations around inner-work for those considering a psychedelic journey or looking to bring more intentionality to their explorations. These are relevant for facilitators as well, as each of us should start with and continue on in our personal healing trajectories.

Journeying Is Work

Medicines can be profound helpers, but they can't do the work for you. Psychedelic experiences can be environments that enable and catalyze more profound inner-work. They can soften our defenses, open our curiosity toward new possibilities, and prompt the broader perspectives that help us not take our attachments so seriously. But consuming a substance does not guarantee these outcomes. They will meet you halfway, and the real work happens in the weeks, months, and years that follow. Decide how much work you are willing and able to do, and remember that pacing is a part of healing. Don't expect to resolve a lifetime of pain and ingrained habits overnight.

Self-awareness gained through journey work can allow you to trace back the roots of your pain and suffering and notice the maladaptive coping strategies you might wish to let go of. Radical healing, healing that gets to the root of things, is a long and courageous road. It often feels like swimming upstream. Set yourself up with the support, breaks, joys, and community needed to engage in this work. Try to see it as part of your life rather than a temporary interruption to it.

Some aspects of our personal healing work can get easier with practice. In my experience, it's the hardest and most cumbersome at the beginning. Access to our innate healing intelligence and magic seems to grow alongside our commitment and the daily choice to stay engaged with the work.

You Won't Always Like It

Inner-work can be gratifying. However, by nature, it is not and should not always be comfortable. If it is, you aren't going deep enough. Self-reflection is inherently vulnerable and bound to be uncomfortable at times. If we are honest with ourselves and invite feedback from others, we will encounter sides of ourselves that are unflattering, surprising, or contradict our ideals. Healing doesn't always mean being the hero of our story; it also means looking at the places where we need to grow or take more responsibility, and the ways we are contributing to our own suffering. This is an opportunity to practice self-compassion and curiosity and steer away from perfectionism and the dreaded shame spiral.

We need to separate the capitalist–wellness complex from our ideas of healing. Be wary of self-help approaches that sell shortcuts, promote benefits that can only be reached through a specific protocol or community, or promise quick fixes to complex problems (and yes, this includes psychedelics). Becoming a more healed, whole, thriving person isn't a product for sale to the highest bidder. It is a unique path each of us must walk, and much of the work happens unglamorously and out of sight.

Instead, keep company with people who normalize personal healing and growth processes. The more we come to see this as a key part of the human experience, the less we will think of it as work, to begin with. Lean on the support of a therapist, counselor, peer support network, partner, coworkers, family, and friends (and know that sometimes, parts of the path are meant to be walked alone).

Some of the discomforts of increasing self-awareness and responsibility can be alleviated through practices such as journaling, somatic activities, artistic self-expression, and spending time in nature. Humor helps a lot too. Lighten up!

Inner-Work Is an Act of Love

We don't just engage in inner-work because it is a "prerequisite" to serve medicine or the right thing to do. That attitude is missing so much. In truth, self-knowledge is an unavoidable part of existing as a conscious being. We have been gifted with a vast capacity for awareness and inherited a profound need to heal. The confluence of the two is inner-work.

It is a path toward intimacy with the one person you'll share your whole life with: you. We can't trade places with anyone else. The pain, gifts, weaknesses, strengths, and unique makeup that we each carry are ours to nurture. Inner-work gives us the opportunity to get to know and love ourselves, not just on the surface level, but the fine details and inner workings.

Self-compassion is central to this work. Even with growing self-awareness, we may act outside of our values when depleted, triggered, or under pressure. Inner-work is not a guarantee that we will always act in alignment with our best selves. It does, however, help us build the capacity to forgive, take accountability, and move forward with lessons learned.

Developing deeper awareness of who you are, what has shaped you, and the parts that need healing can open doors to greater meaning and clarity throughout your life. But more than that, getting to know yourself is an act of love and kindness. It is a form of harm-reduction. It's what each of us can start with to disrupt toxic cycles, create healthier communities, and return to a sustainable world. The curiosity and compassion that begin with ourselves can permeate our relationships and, in some small way, help shape our shared reality in the direction of wholeness.

FOR FACILITATORS

There are other important considerations if you are pursuing the path of a psychedelic facilitator, guide, or therapist.

AWARENESS OF EMOTIONAL LIFE: As a starting point, spend some time reflecting on your relationship with big emotions, uncertain situations, and people you find challenging. What happens within you when confronted with strong emotions? Which ones are you most comfortable or uncomfortable with? Make a list. What situations in your daily life bring out the less-healed parts of you, and how could these surface when working with people in altered states?

What is your attachment style? What is your communication style? How do you respond when you feel surprised, blindsided, accused, uncertain, physically unsafe, emotionally or energetically unequipped? These are all things that can occur in the normal unfolding of a psychedelic experience. Self-knowledge helps us sort through different possible scenarios before we're responsible for someone else and the stakes are high.

PERSONAL PRACTICE: How and when do you set aside time to process the happenings of your life? Do you have daily rituals or a spiritual community? Regardless of secular or spiritual orientation, it is important that we all make a habit of regularly looking inward. This can take different forms. Some people set up an altar or a room in their home where they can meditate, reflect, conduct rituals, offer prayers and intentions, and set down things they wish to let go. Some people participate in religious or community groups that have opportunities for sharing circles and peer support. Others metabolize their life material through expressive means such as dance, sports, arts, writing, land connection, and music.

The key to a personal practice is that it is conscious and intentional. It is about more than feeling good. It requires that we become still enough to listen, reflect, and make meaning from the insights that come to us, and that we have people in our lives who are aware of our growth edges and can support us in enacting the necessary shifts.

SHADOW WHY'S: Whom is your psychedelic service really for—you or your community? We all have conscious and less conscious reasons for wanting to do psychedelic work with others. There are benefits to doing this work, but it's easy for one's reasoning to be muddled. Getting in touch with your "shadow why," as Laura Mae Northrup phrases it in her book *Radical Healership,* is critical for the safety of your clients. Not to eradicate it, but to know it intimately and be prepared to deal with it when it shows up while caring for others.

Concepts such as transcendence and ascension can easily become tools for ego-advancement that do not serve collective healing. Many people come to medicine through their own profound experiences, and in a period of over-identifying with their experiences, rush to wanting to serve medicine. Indeed, becoming guides or leaders in the field when we have not done our inner-work can have serious detrimental effects. This issue is critical enough to merit a whole chapter exploring Shadow. For now, the point is that with the time and maturity that come from conscious self-reflection, life experience, and listening to elders, we can embrace psychedelic medicine as an integral part of our lives rather than allowing it to define us or carry us to an ungrounded, overly invested place.

Community and Supportive Relationships

Our growth and healing do not happen in isolation. We learn about ourselves through interactions with those around us. On the personal and professional levels, community involvement is essential to our health and integrity. Not only can trusting relationships offer reflections that help us see ourselves more clearly and gain self-awareness, but also they are the testing grounds where we work out new ways of being not based on past traumas and triggers. In turn, our immediate communities and most intimate relationships are often the first sites of change that ripples throughout our lives and work.

To be a responsible psychedelic facilitator or field-builder, it is essential to participate in a web of peer support and consultation. Be prepared for your prospective clients to ask you about this, and have an honest answer you can feel good about.

In Conversation with an Elder

I had the honor of speaking with a dear mentor who has been a wellspring of wisdom for me as I've entered this field. For anonymity, we will call her "ML." We discussed mentorship, shadow work, expectations, and preparing for the strangeness of psychedelic states.

"ML" is a psychotherapist, teacher, writer, and healer. For over forty years she has worked with and helped individuals, groups, and communities. Trained in many of the modern psychotherapy techniques and Indigenous healing techniques, ML brings a depth of presence and gentleness to her work with psychedelics, which she began in 2014. She was faculty at a Trauma Studies Program, as well as Columbia

University School of Social Work, the State University of New York, and Mercy College Department of Psychology. She is based in Upstate New York.

RM: *Thank you for taking this time with me. Maybe we could start by exploring what we mean when we say "shadow work," or when we refer to the shadow.*

ML: Before people can be considered for the role of facilitators, they need to spend time doing their own work. Having sat in on a medicine journey, or going to classes—even the fabulous ones—does not train you to serve medicine. Not only do you have to do your own inner-work (so you don't get triggered by the material that's coming up in the person that you're holding space for), but you also have to develop practical skills. Strange things can happen. Are you equipped to sit with that and guide it?

When it comes to choosing a facilitator, one of the things that you can ask is: *What is your relationship with your shadow?* What parts of your psyche have you not explored? What scares you? What are you repelled by? This awareness comes with practice. New sitters, even those with amazing potential, should spend considerable time assisting elders.

RM: *How important do you think it is for sitters to have experience with the medicines?*

ML: If you're going to be a brain surgeon, I don't think you need to have brain surgery. But I think that in holding space, and working with shadows especially, people need to understand the vastness of the inner experience in some of these states. Most people don't know what holding space means.

People who want to facilitate should do a lot of personal inquiry. They need to understand that the work of presence is in many ways a skill of *nondoing.* This is where a lot of people get tripped up. What I call the "fix-it part" comes up. The fix-it part is part of the shadow. *A lot of people want to be helpers. When that part comes up, which is connected with self-validation, that is no longer about presence—it is about satisfying the needs of the sitter.*

Right now, my biggest concern is the number of people who think they can serve medicine. People think that either because it's legal now or because they had a good trip, that means they can serve well. No. That is my biggest concern. Along with the integrity of those who are running training organizations.

The other thing that's coming up for me is that medicine work is not a panacea. Public enthusiasm for this work has literally just mushroomed, right? People who call me and say, "Well, you know, I've been depressed my whole life. So my friend or therapist suggested that I do a journey." And I have to tell them: it's not necessarily going to get rid of your depression, your anxiety, or your PTSD in one session. I think that's part of the shadow of the medicine bubble: that it's being touted as a cure.

I have learned to check in more often with people during their journeys; not to interrupt their processes, but just in case they have a need. Twice, I've had somebody tell me after the fact, "I wish you had checked in." I thought I was respecting their space. So now, I will very gently periodically check in.

It's also important to be clear about the intention for the journey. I'll have people who come to do a journey. And I have people who come specifically to do a piece of therapy work with the support of the medicine. Journey work and psychedelic-assisted therapy are two different things.

RM: *These are two different modalities with very different skills and qualifications involved. The skill of sitting or facilitating can be developed without being a therapist. But people should not be practicing psychotherapy or therapeutic interventions if they are not trained to do that.*

ML: Right. And curing a mental illness is not necessarily the only goal or a useful direction. Unless somebody who's already a therapist is working with somebody who wants to do psychedelic-assisted therapy.

Conclusion

The potential for good and for harm in the emerging psychedelic industries often takes my breath away. So much will be impacted by how community members, leaders, investors, journalists, policymakers, trainers, and facilitators show up in the near future. No problem can be addressed without time spent reflecting and seeking understanding. Without this, we remain in a reactionary place and our solutions will be shaped by that reactivity.

Imagine a society where inner-work is a prioritized, established, and celebrated part of our culture. How might our homes, neighborhoods, organizations, medicine spaces, and communities feel and operate differently? What if we collectively developed intimate self-knowledge that illuminated the ways we've internalized our own oppression, and instead of collapsing in despair, allowed this to activate us toward systemic change, beginning with the things in our realm of control? What if we normalized being aware of our impact on one another and shared a collective investment in finding ways for all of us to thrive?

Perhaps conflicts would not escalate so rapidly into ruptures and harm. Perhaps we would remember that we are held in a web of relationships and change how we are treating our waters, forests, and air. Perhaps we could begin to model at the community level what we wish to see at the societal level: fairness, justice, harmony, and reconciliation. This is the dream that becomes possible on the foundation of inner-work.

CHAPTER 2

Presence

In 2013, I gave birth to my son, Moses. I had gradually come to terms with my loss of faith during my pregnancy. This created space for me to embrace practices that had been deemed "worldly" by the Church. Among them was the practice of mindfulness, which was lumped in with Buddhism, yoga, and a whole array of distinct systems of practice that existed outside of the Judeo-Christian tradition.

I purchased a book called Mindful Birthing that provided me with an inroad to the world of meditation and mindfulness. My husband and I attended birthing classes to prepare. A core message came through repeatedly: presence is central to giving birth. Because it is such an intense somatic, emotional, and spiritual experience, staying in touch and breathing through the present moment can help birth unfold in its natural progression.

I had planned a home birth in my husband's childhood home with the support of a team of midwives from Alma Midwifery. I had been laboring since before sunrise, and by early afternoon I was struggling hard. I was restless and exhausted and began to spend the shortening time between each contraction feeling tense, dreading the next one. I felt like labor was never going to end, and as my internal state began to lock down, so did my body. Progress slowed and I considered transferring to a hospital.

Between health checks, I was sitting in the pool we had set up and I looked up and noticed that our lead midwife was seated on the couch, knitting. She looked relaxed. The other midwife was doing some charting and humming to herself. Meanwhile, I was going through the struggle of my life. At the moment, I felt upset they weren't more actively engaged. "How can they be so calm?" I thought to myself. But what I wanted was for them to take this burden from me, which they couldn't do. Instead, they were intentionally providing me with nonverbal reassurance that this was all a perfectly normal process; there was no emergency or external crisis. They were affirming my ability to get through it.

When I asked for more support, they were responsive and resourced me in changing my environment so I could better face what was coming up. They assisted me in mindfulness exercises, breathwork, and natural relaxation techniques that enabled me to do the work only I could do. They surrounded me and vocalized with me when it came time to push. At a certain point, I had to actively choose to be present and stop *resisting the experience. I had to choose to trust my body, the baby, the intelligence of the natural process, and the skill and expertise of our team. Their role was to ensure my safety, empower me in my process, and bear witness with abiding presence.*

My son was born that evening, at home, perfectly healthy. His name means "drawn from the water." He's a wonder child.

Early on in my labor, I experienced what I later recognized as an expanded state of consciousness. I was lying in my bed as the contractions began to intensify. I could feel an opening in my whole core and let out loud sobs in response. Suddenly, I was transported to a far-off place and could sense the presence of mothers backward and forward in time who had passed through this same initiation. Years later, that day in the treehouse with the mushrooms, I broke down sobbing in a way that was distinctly different from my own voice. I realized I had only heard this once before: the day I was in labor. Those cries had catapulted me into an altered state where I could access the ancestral support I needed. "I've been here before," I thought to myself, and I realized that giving birth and doing journey work have a great deal in common.

Being present in your own psychedelic experience, and facilitating journeys for others, is not so different from supporting someone who is giving birth.

Defining Presence

I define presence as compassionate awareness of this moment. It speaks to radical acceptance of things as they are, rather than preoccupation with how things should be. It anchors itself in what is emerging in real time instead of focusing on what has happened or will happen. Presence is the energy of the witness and the courage to look at what is real. It speaks to a willingness to engage with what is imperfect. In this way, it is linked with harm-reduction, which we will explore at length in its own chapter.

Cultivating the skill of presence helps us build our understanding of the world around us and a grounded sense of our place in it. It asks us to feel and engage our senses, taking in as much information about this moment as is available. With practice, it builds our capacity for being with what is uncomfortable, unknown, and mysterious. When we get still enough to notice, we can become aware.

Presence is more than just "living in the moment," it also means zooming out enough to take a bird's-eye view of our current shared realities. As a matter of fact, radical presence is built off of an understanding of collective history. It means looking with courage at all the moments that have occurred and how they are shaping this present moment. In doing so, we can act from a place of grounded awareness, centered on responsiveness rather than reactivity.

HEALING INTO PRESENCE

Along the healing path, much of our work involves getting in touch with what is keeping us from being present in our lives. Presence enables reconnection. It is not all about sunsets and meditation retreats; it is gritty work that we have to practice day in and day out. We live in a world that offers many enticing distractions and ways to escape our lived reality. These can hold their own value or can make our disconnection worse. Many spiritual traditions teach that reconnecting with our present experience is central to our paths as humans.

Presence takes practice, but it's more than that. The present moment can be difficult, uncomfortable, and even downright unsafe. Humans have powerful and wise survival mechanisms that keep us safe in the face of acute or ongoing trauma. When traumatic experiences occur, this armor protects us from further injury. We need to honor the brilliance and intelligence of this system. However, these adaptations block our ability to be fully present with what is happening in and around us. They can shut out the good along with the bad.

Many times, these initial experiences don't get processed for years, and by then we have adopted habitual strategies that protect us from feeling. I have a loved one who spent several years incarcerated. He has expressed that now, even though his external life has moved forward, his inner world is still caged. He wakes up every morning thinking he is in prison. He has described the resulting numbness that has dulled everything, not just the fear and the pain, but also the joy of watching his child grow up and his connection with those around him. This is a heartbreaking way to live. Repairing this is critical to healing.

This is why developing a trauma-aware practice is so important. We can't muscle our way into embodiment and presence. It is not just about knowledge. It is a process that happens in our bodies and whole selves over time. We must create conditions in which we can gradually unwind our powerful defenses. For many, this means finding spaces that are designed to be "brave spaces" or "safer spaces" in order to relax the nervous system. Engaging the help of a professional (such as a trauma therapist) can be valuable for many people. As is being surrounded by people who have shared language and can walk the path in a peer support context. It takes training, practice, and accountability to work with people who are holding complex trauma.

Exploring Presence

When we embark on our own psychedelic journey work, all of our hopes, fears, and beliefs come with us. Recognizing this material as distinct from external reality frees up our ability to experience the moment and integrate whatever arises. Meditation teachers in the Buddhist tradition say that you are not the thoughts you think. You are the watcher. So in order to be free from attaching to every novel concept or notion that passes through one's awareness during a mushroom trip, for instance, it's important to first become intimately aware of our values, fears, assumptions, and underlying beliefs. This is why a foundation of inner-work is so important for psychedelic journeying.

Awareness and nonattachment are doubly important when we hold space for other people. Not only is their material present in the room, but ours is as well. To hold a supportive container for someone else's healing, we need to know our own material and how it manifests. We need to develop the tools required to set aside or manage internal upsets in real time, so we can effectively show up in service of others. Therapists spend years developing this skill. It takes ongoing awareness, commitment, and practical tools.

FOR JOURNEYERS

As discussed earlier, much of our healing processes involve peeling back the layers of defenses that prevent us from being present. I am not a psychologist, but in my observation, these adaptations can manifest in many ways: unprocessed grief or depression, which keep us locked in a loop of the past, anxiety and fears lodging us in an imagined future, or adaptive mechanisms that armor us from feeling in general through dissociation or numbness. These all pull us out of the present and into internal cages of disconnection.

You have to feel it to heal it.

PREPARATION:　Developing a mindfulness practice is one of the best things you can do to prepare for a psychedelic experience. Months or even years of developing a meditative practice will provide the muscle memory needed to navigate the terrain. The skills are largely the same: noticing, feeling, and allowing. Think back to the birth story from earlier. Similarly, many (but not all) "bad trips" are connected with a person's sense of safety and ability to be present. This isn't a matter of willpower; it is a matter of developing the capacity through repeated practice and experience over time.

Becoming still and quiet enough to set clear intentions is another key part of the preparation, and this process is only possible through presence with your needs, desires, and motivations.

DURING AND AFTER:　During your psychedelic experience, see if you can take the experience one breath at a time. It will likely unfold and evolve in unexpected ways. Think of it like riding waves, and be open to surprises. Bracing for unknowns or guarding against what we fear might come up is a recipe for a difficult experience. Talk with your facilitator about any concerns you have and strategies you can turn to if and when presence becomes difficult.

See if you can notice, without naming or analyzing, the experience as it unfolds. Resist the impulse to talk. Your facilitator can take notes on things shared during the session that you'd like to revisit later. But it's beneficial to not get swirled up into interpretation in real time, as you may miss important experiences and insights as they play out. Practice turning your attention toward what you are feeling, sensing, and experiencing.

FOR FACILITATORS

Check in with your scope of practice. What kind of training have you had surrounding trauma, somatics, and mindfulness? What kinds of clients are you qualified, or unqualified, to work with? Take steps to form a referral network of facilitators you can turn to when you meet prospective clients who are outside of your scope.

The practice of mindfulness and deep awareness is foundational to holding space for others. The more we develop the ability to notice what is arising in the moment without needing to react or change it, the better equipped we will be to create space for our clients' emergent experience.

Being responsive to the journeyer's needs and experience depends on your ability to be present. Presence is needed for the complex task of tracking your experience, the experience of the journeyer, and the larger environment and safety considerations. In addition to being present and aware, facilitators also need to be able to regulate themselves. The more you can notice what is happening around and within you, the more responsive you can be and the more grounded decisions you can make in real time.

SELF-AWARENESS: All of our explorations of inner-work and discernment come together in the present moment. This is where we take what we have learned and integrate and apply it to our lives and work. The benefits of inner-work show up in the room. You have to prepare long before you're in the room holding space for someone.

ABIDING PRESENCE: With a nondirective approach, the role of the facilitator is to create and protect space. To tend the container. This does *not* just mean sitting silently in the room and making sure they don't trip while walking to the bathroom. This is an energetic guarding that can have deep significance, depending on what philosophy the facilitator and client are coming from. It means finding ways to convey compassion, care, and goodwill, not just through words, but through body language, energy, and the way you tend the space.

TRACKING: As you navigate a session with a client, your ability to track their experience, cues, and emotional and energetic shifts will all play a role in how you hold space for them as a facilitator. In tandem with this, you will need to be tracking your own experience. This is why presence requires practice—it is a skill of relaxed awareness. Think of the difference between focused vision and relaxed vision. When holding space for someone, you need to engage in relaxed awareness. This means being able to take in many kinds of sensory information at once. What is being said? What is my client's body language communicating? How are my body and mind feeling at this moment? What is arising for my client? What is arising for me? What is happening in the environment that might be impacting the experience? Does anything need to change? Why am I talking? Why am I touching?

ATTUNEMENT: As discussed in chapter 9, on Consent, the ability to tune in to another person's experience is central to holding space. This involves witnessing, caring, and allowing yourself to feel what they are expressing and signaling. From there, respond appropriately and take necessary action so your client feels as supported and empowered as possible. In some ways, this means softening the boundaries between yourself and your client, without losing your professional footing. It is a high-level skill to soften enough to really tune in while staying grounded enough in your experience and your duties as the facilitator. These blurry boundaries are one reason facilitators do not consume the medicines when they are holding space, and why we work in consultation with peers to process sessions after they take place.

STANDING GUARD: To some, entheogens are portals into other realms. The facilitator's role is to stand guard at the gate and welcome the journeyer back upon their return. They provide an anchor to consensus reality and assure the journeyer that they can venture out and come through to the other side. To facilitate literally means to create ease. So we are not doing the work or guiding the work. We are doing our part to smooth the path for the person we are serving. This means creating comfortable conditions, providing encouragement and reassurance, as well as reaffirming the client with kindness and unconditional positive regard.

WHAT CAN ARISE: Presence is not just about support and care. It is also a safeguard so that when things are not going right, you have the ability to notice early on and course correct. Difficult energies can emerge during psychedelic sessions. Two common instances are transference and erotic energy. Even for those who are not psychologists or therapists, a baseline understanding of projection and transference can be helpful, since they happen around us and between us all the time.

Projection is when a person attributes one's own traits or experiences onto someone else. A simple example could be when someone says their child or pet is anxious when it is actually they themselves who are feeling anxious.

Relatedly, transference happens when a person directs the feelings or desires they hold for a key figure in their life onto another person (in this case, the facilitator). Once, I was trip-sitting for my best friend and she said, "I feel like you're my mom." This is an obvious example of transference. She went on to share how she felt inadequate and like she would never measure up to my standards for her. I am not a therapist, so I was in no position to interpret her statement; in fact, it brought up my own triggers around our relationship that I had to manage. This type of transference is common during psychedelic experiences, and it can be especially tricky in dual relationships. We spent some time processing this later when she was in a sober state.

In addition to the transference that can happen between a client and facilitator, there can also be mutual attraction and erotic energy that arises. *It is unethical to have sexual contact with a client at any time, especially while they are in an altered state.* As such, it is important to acknowledge that this attraction can occur so it does not catch you off-guard. Denial of these dynamics perpetuates shame and secrecy, and does not serve the goals of ethical practice. Forces of attraction can be powerful and intoxicating, and facilitators are vulnerable to ethical breaches if they don't have a plan ahead of time for how to handle them. Spend some time in peer support contexts (and on your own) working through scenarios of what could happen in a session. Make a plan for the steps you can take to protect your client and yourself from getting into a compromising situation. If you are aware of an existing attraction between you and a prospective client, refer them to someone else who can provide them with the level of energetically clear support that they need. If a line is crossed, consult with a peer or mentor as soon as possible in order to get support in addressing the situation.

In Conversation with Gillian Scott-Ward, PhD

I had the pleasure of meeting Gillian at a New York gathering to uplift Black voices and culture makers in psychedelics. The event was organized by our mutual friend and trusted colleague, Victor Cabral, who is interviewed in chapter 5, on Community. I was struck by the depth of insights Gillian offered and the way she continuously centered the body and the spirit in her remarks about this sacred work. We met to discuss presence, nature connection, and ritual.

Gillian Scott-Ward, PhD (Cornell, BA 2004, City University of New York, PhD, 2011) is an internationally recognized clinical psychologist, filmmaker, Reiki practitioner, and advocate for social justice. She specializes in healing through the mind-body-soul connection, integrating culturally relevant psychodynamic thought with Eye Movement Desensitization and Reprocessing (EMDR) therapy, mindfulness-based stress reduction, and energy psychology. She is a graduate of the Psychedelic-Assisted Therapies and Research Certificate program at the California Institute of Integral Studies and currently practices Ketamine-Assisted Psychotherapy (KAP) with an emphasis on connecting clients with the healing potential of ancestral wisdom.

RM: *Can we start by talking about what presence means in the work that you do with your clients?*

GSW: People come to me because they yearn for something different. More often than not, something in their life feels out of alignment. It can feel overwhelming to know you want change, and not know how or where to begin. I have come to believe that for many, an important first step to living in alignment—with intention—is to cultivate presence. That is, to cultivate compassionate, nonjudgmental, and curious awareness. To increase our observing ego, which is our ability to zoom out and gain perspective and distance from what is happening at any given moment. This enables us to see the bigger picture so that we can respond intentionally rather than reacting to all the stimuli that are happening around us and inside of us all the time. This can help us be creators in our lives—instead of feeling stuck.

Psychedelics can come into the picture as we work with people to develop rituals and practices that expand one's ability to have presence during a regular day. But there can be barriers to developing presence.

So often, what I see in my work is a chronic biological stress response. When I first meet with someone, I take time to learn about their experiences—what it feels like to live in their bodies, what their relationships are like, and what their spiritual life is like. It has been helpful for people to understand the interplay between the body and mind. Early on in my therapeutic relationships, I show people a diagram about the impact of stress on the body. The impact of what many people experience as chronic hypervigilance. This nebulous, constant feeling of waiting for the other shoe to drop. So many times, people look at the diagram and have "aha" moments like, "My dentist did tell me it looked like I was grinding my teeth. . . . I guess it could be stress." They may begin to attune to the fact that their chronic neck pain, headaches, stomach issues, sex drive, heart palpitations, and trouble breathing aren't "just the way they are" but rather signals from their body to be paid attention to, respected, and addressed. That the body carries wisdom and awareness. The problem is, so many of us are rewarded for ignoring our body cues, inner-knowing, and spiritual wisdom. Cultivating presence helps us regain these vital skills for an aligned life.

I practice in New York City. So even the energy of the city can make us feel "always on," always vigilant, always needing to do or achieve, which can be counter to cultivating presence. Sometimes our experiences in early life can make it really difficult to be present. Maybe we're worried about our safety, whether it's psychological or physical. Maybe we become overly attuned to people's responses to us and instead of being connected to our inner-experience, we become more connected to other people's experiences of us. Add factors related to our identities, specifically marginalized or systematically oppressed identities, and we may find that this constant vigilance, anxiety, or disconnection from our authentic selves felt necessary for survival. All of those things can make it very difficult to be present. This can lead us to develop rigid patterns of thinking, behaving, and experiencing the world for survival—which impedes our ability to thrive authentically. And so even when we work very hard on practices and rituals to get present, there could be this ceiling, a limit to how much shift we can make on our own.

When I began working clinically with ketamine I realized, combined with other rituals and practices, we could amplify change in people's bodies—allowing them to connect with curious awareness and nonjudgment. Practices I was already using in therapy like mindfulness, meridian tapping, movement, and connection to nature had their effects amplified when used with KAP. Rituals, practices, and behaviors were more easily helping my clients shift their energetic and bodily states. So, I believe that plant medicine or psychedelic medicine can really help make change and break through barriers that may prevent people from being really present. But it's not just the medicine—it's a medicine in addition to these practices.

RM: *Do you think there are specific practices that can help us tap into that awareness, and maybe even quiet some of the noise to sense the subtler things?*

GSW: Absolutely. I practice therapy in nature. Even though I'm sort of in the middle of New York City. With the pandemic, my in-person sessions are largely in the Park, near water, in nature. We start and end all of our sessions practicing awareness and connection to the nature around us. We know for a fact that being in a forest around nature lowers the stress response and allows us to be present. You can't be present in a constant chronic state of fight or flight. So rituals that help to quiet the nervous system, to be still, and to turn down the thoughts are really important and really helpful.

So, having a nature practice is really foundational. Doing breathwork. Spending time learning and understanding how the central nervous system works. It's really important to understand how the body responds to threats, and find individual ways to manage that. Anything that connects body movement and breath can be really helpful. I think similar to ketamine, there are other realms of goodness, stability, and calm that you can feel in your body. Folks may need some support to access it. How can you know if you're there, or if you're getting there, if you've never experienced it before?

In Conversation with Andre Humphrey

Andre Humphrey is the founder of Inner City Bliss, a 501(c)3 nonprofit working with schools and organizations across the Bay Area, with the mission of providing resources and support to Black and brown communities living in the inner city. Andre is trained in trauma-informed holistic wellness practices. He completed his Yoga Instructor E-RYT 300 from Aura Wellness, as well as the Trauma Informed Training from Niroga Institute. He has been practicing these techniques for over a decade and has used them to aid his own healing journey from childhood trauma. His goal is to make the life-transforming tools of meditation and yoga accessible to inner cities all over the world. Andre is also a student mentor at Alma Institute and helped shape the curriculum for Alma's Psilocybin Facilitator Certificate program.

RM: *How important is it for people to pace themselves when working with psychedelics and plant medicines?*

AH: Well, I think the most important thing to understand is that healing takes time. The psychedelic sacraments are not a one-stop, one-ceremony, fix-your-life type of thing. Most of us have dealt with trauma or even just the pain of living in these bodies in this lifetime. We establish all these mental patterns, negative thinking, and emotional patterns.

Unraveling those unhealthy thinking patterns, emotional patterns, and living patterns can take time. So when we understand that healing is a process with its own timeline, we can accept that it's not possible to unwind everything at once. When it comes to the sacraments, if you're engaging with them properly, then you're spending a good amount of time in preparation before and integration afterward. Ideally, there is quite a bit of time put into preparing. It could mean changing your diet, focusing on your intentions, and organizing your life to support a big experience. The same thing is true with integration, if you're taking time to integrate your experiences, that could take a week, a month, or even a lifetime—depending on which sacrament you're working with. So in my humble opinion, pacing comes from doing it properly. And if we're preparing and integrating properly, that'll naturally put us in a position where we're having to pace ourselves instead of jumping from one psychedelic experience to the next.

RM: *How do you see mindfulness and trauma healing as being connected?*

AH: Well, when we experience trauma, these experiences affect our thinking patterns. They affect our emotional patterns. They affect how we feel in our bodies. And mindfulness is this present moment awareness. It requires slowing down enough to become aware of these reactive thinking patterns. Aware of my emotional patterns. Aware of how these patterns are making me feel in my body. So through becoming aware, we can learn how to see our experiences through a different lens and take steps to move beyond those patterns toward wholeness and well-being.

I think mindfulness practices play a major role in all of this, from preparation through integration. Learning how to be present, learning how to breathe through challenging experiences, learning how to be aware of your thoughts, and how they make you feel in your body. Those are valuable skills to develop, whether you're preparing for a journey or integrating one. In my humble opinion, mindfulness is actually one of the best practices to prepare you for a psychedelic journey, and it also helps you integrate the messages that you receive.

When you take a psychedelic, you're going to be in that space for an enhanced period of time. You really want to develop the skill of being comfortable in stillness, being with your breath, and being with your thoughts. Being comfortable with discomfort, surrender, and patience. I also believe a lot of the really difficult psychedelic experiences can be connected to not being prepared mentally, emotionally, and spiritually with your intentions, or not being prepared with the skills needed to ride the waves of the experience. If you're not comfortable in that space of surrender and awareness, then psychedelic journeys can be very challenging.

RM: *Are there things you have learned through that work that have surprised you?*

AH: I think the biggest thing that I've learned is that trauma is real. Those experiences you had in your childhood or in your adulthood: those things are real. And they show up in experiences in every aspect of your life. Everybody's dealing with trauma to varying degrees. It's common for people who are coming to recognize the weight of things they've lived through to feel like a victim, and that no one can relate to your pain. Through doing this work with people on a larger scale, I have realized that everybody's dealing with trauma on some level.

RM: *How does trauma-informed care apply to working with psychedelics?*

AH: As a facilitator, I need to first be aware of my own traumas and shadows so that I know what I may be bringing into the space. So if anything comes up or triggers me, I can notice what I'm moving through and how I'm showing up with that. It also means becoming skilled enough to hold space for others' trauma responses without taking things personally, or getting emotionally attached to a specific healing outcome. Being trauma-informed requires us to consider how the environment we create can support people in being safe enough to participate, and knowing they bring their history in with them. It requires creating choices and checking in so people feel they can participate within their limits. Even though we all have trauma, working with trauma requires skills and training because a lot can come up.

RM: *How do you take care of yourself, especially after experiences where you've been witnessing someone's trauma?*

AH: The number-one thing that I do after any kind of intense energetic exchange is cleansing my space. Then, I sit in meditation and try to go over my memory of the experience from a nonattached place. Almost like I'm watching a movie and I'm seeking perspective on how I could have shown up differently, stronger, or pulled back a bit. So I actually physically cleanse the space, make time to sit with the experience, and take in all the lessons I can learn from it. I practice this repeatedly, so I can show up better and be more supportive in future experiences.

Conclusion

Presence is a gift of consciousness. For many of us, it has been compromised or taken away by the forces of struggle and oppression. Presence is precious, hard-earned, and imperfect. It often takes years to cultivate, and by definition, there is no such thing as an arrival. Every small step toward allowing yourself to feel is a kindness to yourself and others.

When you find moments where you are present, relish in them. Let your body and nervous system enjoy how good it can feel. You are alive. You're able to access awareness, sensation, calm, pleasure, and even pain and discomfort. You are noticing. You are here. You are participating in this moment. Remind your precious system that this is possible and worth practicing, and reward yourself for the courage. Surround yourself with people who value presence too.

CHAPTER 3

Shadow

When I was in high school, I enrolled in every art class offered. I loved drawing, painting, sculpture, and graphic design. One of the culminating projects in my painting class was a large self-portrait that was representative of my inner world. I had no idea how to convey the conflicted inner world I knew intimately. After a few days' reflection and a bin full of discarded sketches, I finally drew a faceless version of myself standing in my school hallway, divided straight down the middle.

One side of my body held light iridescent colors and symbols of purity, wholesomeness, and life: flowers, waterfalls, keys, books, stars, and Christian symbols. To me, these were the aspects of myself that were acceptable and "good." Predictably, the other side held the darker aspects. My insides were shrouded in gray and black and enclosed by a gate overgrown with brambles. Behind the gate lay crows and spiderwebs (which I now venerate) alongside imagery that suggested death, heartbreak, sex, and rebellion. I associated this side with my doubts about my religion, the trauma of sexual assaults I had experienced, and the grief over two friends lost to suicide. Entire parts of myself had gotten tangled up in the mess of it all, and I didn't know how to get them back.

This polarity was something that intensified throughout my adolescence. Every weekend, I found myself on stage at church leading worship for a large congregation. At night, I was sneaking through my window and driving out of town with my "bad" friends to get stoned as a break from the pressure and confusion. Because I didn't have a singular place I could fully exist, I developed a fractured sense of self. I had rejected entire parts of myself, with the greatest casualties being my sexuality, vulnerability, and fascination and trust for altered states.

It wasn't until a decade later, when I shook my life loose and embarked on a healing process with psilocybin mushrooms, that I began to integrate into my whole self. I had to knock down many parts of my life—my belief system, my marriage, my career—and do the slow work of rebuilding. This required a great deal of grief, unlearning, and parts work; I had to excavate the parts of myself that I had repressed and illuminate them. I had to do a lot of biographical work to understand when I had departed from myself and why. Then I had to repair those initial wounds that told me the only way to be safe and loved was to eradicate the unacceptable.

It's work that continues. Thankfully, the mushrooms have taught me a great deal about the beauty in the dark—those depths hold the potential for a rich life and transformation. Mushrooms have taught me that the forces of life and death, order and chaos, and harm and healing are inseparable from one another and exist in mysterious, dynamic, and ongoing cycles. This is the alchemical magic of shadow work.

Defining Shadow

Shadow can be defined as the unconscious, wounded, or rejected parts of ourselves and our movements. It is the "other side of the coin." Often, shadow is out of alignment with shared or collective values, so it remains out of sight, unacknowledged, and can take on a life of its own.

The original concept of the shadow self was popularized by Swiss psychiatrist Carl Jung. In 1938, he wrote:

> Unfortunately there can be no doubt that man is, on the whole, less good than he imagines himself or wants to be. Everyone carries a shadow, and the less it is embodied in the individual's conscious life, the darker and denser it is. If an inferiority is conscious, one always has a chance to correct it. . . . But if it is repressed and isolated from consciousness, it never gets corrected.[1]

We all have shadows, and they're often directly tied with our gifts and strengths. When discussing the shadow, I often think of an epic tale where a character reaches a crossroads and they must decide how to use their powers. Some choose expressions that are good and helpful while others choose self-serving and harmful expressions. While life isn't actually that binary, it might be helpful to recognize that shadows are aspects of ourselves, not simply flaws or weaknesses.

Shadow aspects can also be understood as imbalances: unhealed trauma, ancestral burdens, unexamined parts of ourselves, and flaws that have been buried beneath shame and fear. We all have parts of ourselves that we embrace and others that we reject. Polarity is part of being alive, and many philosophers have stated that there would be no beauty, life, or joy without their contrasting counterparts. If we attempt to eradicate the "negative" aspects, we simply shrink the relative range of possibility. By playing this whack-a-mole game of denial and erasure, we don't actually free ourselves from what we are avoiding; new versions of that polarity will continuously form to take their place. What if, instead, we embraced our shadows as teachers?

Often, the people around us will identify our shadows before we do, because others are impacted by the shadows we cast. This is why we have spent so much time discussing awareness thus far. In order to move with clarity and integrity in our personal lives while holding space for others, we need to be conscious of our whole selves.

Parts work (such as Internal Family Systems) enables us to hold awareness of many parts of ourselves at once. These various parts have different needs, desires, motives, and origination points. As we get to know these parts, we can become more intimately aware of and compassionate toward our shadow selves. Through this, we gain experience. This skill can expand from the personal to the world. It can free us of binary thinking and make space for the contradictions inherent to life.

Developing a skill set for working with the shadow in ways that are both curious and compassionate is important for your own medicine work, as well as serving and holding space for others. Your beliefs about shadow will directly impact the way you perceive healing.

Exploring Shadow

While the experience of all-encompassing love and light can be beautiful parts of our experience of life, this is not the full picture. Leaning into "love and light-ism" or "good vibes only" as a way of life is an incomplete approach that runs the risk of perpetuating harm by not acknowledging the difficult realities of the world or the ways that our privilege and use of power contribute to them. This is also known as toxic positivity.

Repression happens when we deny inherently human parts of ourselves. When we repress our shadows, difficult emotions, or negative thoughts, those aspects of ourselves don't just disappear. They find ways to surface. Instead of seeking to eradicate the parts of ourselves or the world that we're uncomfortable with, there's another option. It is possible to "vibrate higher"—to live in alignment with a worldview centered on love and harmony—in a way that is grounded in our collective realities. We can set out to continuously align with the highest good for all—and this path contains not only love and light, it also holds compassion, healing, justice, and action.

Light and shadow are not mutually exclusive. As Daoist philosophy so beauti-fully reflects with its concepts of yin/yang, they are inextricably bound up in one another. As a pertinent example, the global awareness of psilocybin *velada* cere-monies held a shadow of the harm done to María Sabina and the community of Huautla de Jiménez, which we'll discuss in a future chapter. The shadow of legaliza-tion of psychedelics is the resulting commodification of them entering a capitalist market. The shadow of receiving cosmic insights might be a resulting inflation of the ego that then must be managed. The shadow of a nurturing psychedelic facilitator may be their deeply felt desire to be needed. The shadow of an individualistic journeyer's work could be their impulse to use new insights in pursuit of self-advancement and further participation in destructive systems.

COLLECTIVE SHADOW WORK

Shadow doesn't just exist on an individual level; it exists in our families, societies, and the planet as a whole. Our individual work is a microcosm of what needs to happen collectively, and urgently, if we are to course-correct from this self-destructive path humanity is on.

When applied in a broader sense, shadow speaks to the unintended impacts of our systems and our impulses to reject what we fear or don't understand. The hunger for power and wealth is often the shadow expression of a fear of vulnerability, loss of connection, or lack of belonging. It is the move from a prosocial to an antisocial way of being.

The most obvious examples are the ways fear and distrust of each other have festered for generations as war, racism, sexism, homophobia, transphobia, ableism, and ecological destruction—along with so many other expressions of violence. Even our cultural associations equating light with good and dark with evil carry problematic connotations that perpetuate distrust of dark-skinned people. These are the things we need to examine. Collective shadow work means moving beyond the symptoms to the heart of the shadow and seeking to understand and heal it at the root. *In this way, shadow work is transformative justice work.*

We can see poignant examples of collective shadow work from around the world. Consider Germany, which continues to pay billions in restitution to victims of the Holocaust and their families. Importantly, they have also integrated a critical analysis of history into their educational curriculum. Consider also South Africa's Truth and Reconciliation Commission, created to address the violence and injustices that occurred during apartheid. While imperfect answers, the act of publicly telling the truth about history and taking steps to be accountable is an example of collective shadow work. The United States has yet to take meaningful action toward accountability and repair for the enslavement of African American communities and the displacement and genocide of Indigenous communities.

THE COST OF AVOIDING THE SHADOW

Connected to what we discussed in chapter 1, on Inner-Work, engaging with the shadow is inherently uncomfortable. There is a reason our psyches choose to repress certain difficult emotions or parts of ourselves we don't feel free to embrace or trust.

We are in a period of history that requires majorly uncomfortable shifts to more humane and sustainable ways of living together on this planet. That is what is at stake during our lifetimes. This is stated without an ounce of hyperbole: continued collective denial will result in our demise. In the immediate term, denial of our shadows means embracing a death culture. It condones the daily carrying out of physical, cultural, and economic violence and injustice that has been normalized. It leaves us so dissociated from reality that we are willing to look the other way while we bulldoze a football field's worth of old-growth Amazon forest every day to extract profits from the land. It means armoring our tender parts so that we can cope with the desecration of sacred waters and lives and land. It means resigning ourselves to a gradual and very painful unraveling that is completely preventable, impacting the most marginalized and oppressed communities first.

Reckoning with our collective shadows is life-saving work at a global species level.

Shadow in the Medicine Space

In Kylea Taylor's book, *The Ethics of Caring*, she describes shadow "not as the *opposite* of some quality, but rather the *same* quality, one which is expressed as *not enough or too much*."[2] On one side of the spectrum is the insufficient expression of a quality due to fear, while on the other side is an excess due to desire or longing.

From this outlook, Kylea lays out an insightful framework called the Chart of Professional Ethical Vulnerabilities, wherein the center line demonstrates the balance of a quality, and on either side are the shadow manifestations, with fears, desires, and longings. Her book is a defining work on the topic of shadow within altered states work and should be considered required reading for anyone working in this field.

While we can't eradicate our relationships with forces like love, insight, sex, or money (Taylor lists seven core centers), we do have a responsibility to find centered relationships with them in order to not project our shadows onto our clients. This imbalance of expression is where the harm from the shadow self can occur, and the dissolution of boundaries makes it apparent why working with people in altered states presents such vulnerabilities.

I have chosen not to divide this section into lists for facilitators and seekers. The manifestation of shadow occurs in ways that are endlessly universal and individual, so it seems better for us all to reflect together on how shadow manifests itself in both our personal and professional lives.

PSYCHEDELIC SHADOWS

Stanislav Grof coined the term *nonspecific amplifier* to describe the effect psychedelics can have on the state of the person who ingests them. In other words, these powerful substances can turn up the volume on all kinds of material, including detrimental as well as beneficial thoughts, beliefs, and inner states. Here are a few of the most common shadows I've encountered in the medicine space.

SPIRITUAL BYPASSING: A way of avoiding discomfort or pain by applying a spiritual wash over one's difficulties. This is a common and convenient tactic in the psychedelic world, and it's not always done consciously. It carries within it a desire to "skip to the end"—to leap to a position of harmony glimpsed in altered states, without acknowledging the great disharmony we are currently experiencing. It seeks to exist in a place of insulated peace without addressing the discord we are inflicting on one another and the planet. It seeks to embrace love and light without creating space for the shadows that give them form.

PSYCHEDELIC ESCAPISM: The temptation to exist in the world of altered states. It is understandable, especially when it provides us respite from the dire state of the modern world. Escapism can be good medicine in certain moments. It allows us a chance to rest, feel joy, and access a sense of connectedness and peace. It can refill us with strength and grace to carry on in our daily lives. If we make a habit of checking out of the present to exist in other realities, there is a risk of disengaging from our full lives and relationships and developing a preference for altered states.

NARCISSISM: For years, the dominant narrative within psychedelic communities was that psychedelic substances could occasion what is known as "ego death." This experience, reported by people who consume psilocybin mushrooms, DMT, or other substances, can produce feelings of oneness, unity consciousness, total loss of self, and dissolution of boundaries between self and other.

Having experienced this myself (catalyzed by an unassuming teapot full of *cyanescens* mushrooms), I can attest that ego dissolution can be a profound and life-altering experience . . . if integrated in a meaningful way. On the other hand, there is also the potential that these temporary experiences of oneness can actually inflate or reinforce a person's ego upon their return to "default reality."

There has been an important concern in recent years around the intersection of psychedelics, narcissistic personalities, and cult dynamics. This has come in response to an increasing number of allegations of abuse and misuse of power by therapists in both the underground and aboveground psychedelic healing contexts. The emergence of these situations (many of which played out for years without being addressed) has brought into question the previous notion that psychedelics had mitigating effects on egocentric personality traits.

In 2022, two leaders in the field, Emma Knighton, LCPC, and Hannah McLane, MD, presented a talk hosted by Chacruna Institute exploring these intersections.[3] In their talk, they explain that all people exhibit narcissistic personality traits at times throughout their lives. Emma compassionately explained one theory about how Narcissistic Personality Disorder (NPD) often forms early in childhood as a response to adverse or traumatic events marked by shame and neglect. A result is a person who holds an extreme need for validation from others and is highly sensitive to criticism or rejection. These people are often very charming and charismatic, and on the flip side, can have a major need to maintain power and control over others as a means to feel secure. The amplifying qualities of psychedelic experiences can be enticing for people who have narcissistic traits, or NPD, because they affirm their ideas about themselves and the world.

Other Vulnerabilities

In addition to the above, psychedelics can be nonspecific amplifiers and can lower our usual defenses. This means there is less holding back of expressions of shadow in psychedelic spaces. We must tread lightly, work in community, and be willing to notice, name, and tend to one another's blind spots when they arise. Current and past manifestations of shadow in the psychedelic space include:

- Cult dynamics
- Sexual and romantic entanglements within therapeutic relationships
- Cultural theft, biopiracy, and other colonial and extractive practices
- Facilitators serving medicine to meet a personal need (i.e., financial, emotional, and spiritual)
- Self-optimization and biohacking (i.e., "how microdosing can make you a better capitalist")
- Corporatization, patent overreach, and the drive to make rich people richer
- Attempted mind control experiments such as MK-Ultra

- The history of research without consent, especially on marginalized and imprisoned populations
- Paternalistic or fear-based attitudes that we must limit or control access to psychedelic substances

Paired with a highly individualistic society in which this work is reemerging, it makes sense that we're seeing such an overlap between spiritual bypassing, escapism, narcissism, and cult-like dynamics. Instead of demonizing people who exhibit any of these traits, we may first recognize the ways these same traits manifest in our own lives and work to get to the root of those behaviors. Second, we can learn to recognize the signs and behaviors of these shadows and establish boundaries to protect ourselves and our communities from problematic power dynamics. We'll discuss Power at length in chapter 6.

Reflections for All of Us

- What do I already know about my shadow?
- In what ways might my strengths and gifts express themselves as shadow sides?
- Whom can I count on to give me honest and direct feedback when I need it?
- Have people pointed out my blind spots before? Are there patterns in this feedback?
- When is the last time I heard something I believed to be true, but was unwilling or unable to accept?
- What inconvenient or uncomfortable parts of life do I prefer not to engage with?
- What injustices do I look away from because they are intolerable?
- What might be the inherited or cultural shadow in my family line?
- What might healing or loving my shadows look like for me?

In Conversation with June, a Mentor and Underground Psychedelic Guide

There are few people I have seen modeling healthy relationships with shadow in practice. "June" is someone I admire for her ability to hold the shadow with deep compassion and curiosity. I have learned a great deal from her about "both/and" thinking, which is the capacity to hold a great many things to be true at once. It was an honor to speak with her for this book.

June works with people who are integrating psychedelic medicines into their healing journeys. With a special interest in ancestral/generational trauma and complex PTSD, her work is driven by a desire to help people feel safe and fundamentally worthy. In addition to her work with individuals, she strives to create a safe, nurturing, and resilient culture of healing around the integration of psychedelic medicines into modern society. She sees the potential and realizes the interconnectedness of our personal healing with collective liberation. She has been doing anti-oppression, equity, and access work in the psychedelic community since 2018.

RM: *What do you see as the importance of the underground, also known as the grassroots community, particularly when so much is happening in policy change?*

June: For me, the important thing that's happening is that we are grappling with the real questions of what ethics and accountability look like in practice. When we step outside of structured systems, definitions change because we don't have established channels for upholding standards. When we're talking about what safety means, for example, in the context of legalization or a highly regulated field, we're often talking about how to avoid litigation. But in practice, the question of safety runs deeper. We have to really work with each other around what it means to be safe people, safe facilitators, safe practitioners, and safe colleagues. That conversation is very different from just avoiding legal risk.

When it comes to ethics, we're grappling with the question of how to meet a client's needs and preferences with regard to touch. Part of the question is, what do the people seeking healing actually need? Human beings are hardwired for physical connection as a means of coregulating and increasing feelings of worthiness. So oftentimes what's needed is safe touch. This means nonsexual touch that is decided upon between a facilitator and a client *before going into a session* when the client is able to give sober consent. In the underground, there are opportunities for a lot more nuance and case-by-case decision-making, which really honors the individual and honors our humanity in a different way. There's something that happens in medicalization or clinicalization—something gets lost there. At the same time, we have to think about whether or not we're offering something in the realm of touch that is outside of our scope of training.

RM: *What if these practices aren't inherently safer and more ethical in one setting or another? What if the amount of regulation just shapes how much possibility and capacity there are? And with less regulation comes risks, and, I would venture, more potential benefits.*

June: Totally. The underground is not at all unique in being full of people who cause harm, and who are unsafe and unethical. That's a human problem. Having a license or being insured absolutely does not mean that you're a safe facilitator. A shocking percentage of licensed therapists have sexual relationships with their clients. And it's not just psychedelic therapy. We need to admit that it is a fantasy that legal or aboveground is inherently safe.

Yet we demonize the underground. If you zoom out enough, you really have to contend with the lack of logic. It makes me wonder, where are we making decisions from, if they're not coming from logic and reason? Are they based on fear? Are they based on control? Are they based on maintaining power?

Along those lines, Leia Friedwoman, "The Psychedologist," is creating this colored flag system that several of us are collaborating on. It's really, really good. This is to empower the public. To help them see what they should be looking for in a facilitator, and distill it down into simple green, yellow, orange, or red flags.

Relatedly, if white facilitators are operating without an acknowledgment of their privilege or without doing something in the realm of creating access and safety for BIPOC facilitators and clients, aren't we just replicating the same systems of oppression we're giving lip service to healing from?

We're trying to create and nurture something precious here. And it's not just getting started either. We're talking about centuries of these practices. There are parallels to underground abortion, death with dignity, you know; within movements there have been people who are working with a ton of integrity and moving from a place of their morality and ethics, as opposed to waiting for permission from systems that have only ever harmed. And we have such a debt of gratitude to so many, going centuries back, and also our elders right now who never stopped working. Even in the face of prohibition.

RM: *I'm wondering, beyond the obvious major abuses of power or consent violations, how else do you think shadow is manifesting in the movements we are a part of within the psychedelic field?*

June: I think there are a lot of "shadow whys." In Laura Mae Northrup's book, *Radical Healership,* she references the shadow whys, the unconscious motives for what we do. We have to look at the reasons why we're doing things that are not necessarily coming from a place of clean energy. They may be coming from a place of trauma, shame, or self-service. This is why we talk about making sure that facilitators are staying in the work of their own healing. So that we do less of that. Because it can manifest with clients and within the community in all kinds of ways. There's a lot of psychedelic transference that happens, that I think a lot of facilitators kind of feed off of.

The medicine can put people in this state of cosmic openness. And often-times, people have these incredible experiences of self-love, especially when we're working with MDMA. It can be this experience of having one's authen-tic self in the driver's seat for several hours. Deep listening and relationship can happen in that space. There can be this sense that the person holding that space is doing something really special. It's very typical for clients to become kind of enamored and gushy with the facilitator.

I believe for a lot of people who have moved into medicine work without really spending time doing their own work kind of glom onto that feeling. They want to believe it. They need to feel like there's something special about them. And yes, maybe they're able to hold a really nice space. But people conflate their experience with the medicine with the person who is holding space for them. And some facilitators can really internalize that praise.

RM: *Do you have a sort of set philosophy or approach that you take with dual relationships?*

June: This is an area that I've been growing into where my boundaries need to be. I feel like it's a huge responsibility to be someone who is holding space for people's healing. I don't want to confuse the dynamic in any way or poten-tially interrupt their process by having my clients emotionally show up for me. This isn't to say you can't have a very sweet collaborative relationship with a lot of love. This work isn't totally one-sided. The real distinction is that when you're in that facilitator role for someone, not only does that take precedence, but it really fills the whole space of the relationship. Whatever is being done in that relationship should be in service of their healing, growth, whatever they've come to you for and asked you to hold space for.

And then when there's conflict, all of a sudden the person who's the facilitator or the teacher is always going to have more power in that dynamic. That person gets to choose if there's a conflict. They get to ask themselves, "Am I engaging with you as your friend? Or am I going to exert my power over you as your teacher and as knowing more than you do?" It's a very real risk.

RM: *Is there anything we haven't touched on that feels important to discuss?*

June: Another important thing that's happening in the underground is a lot of conversation and effort around the culture that's being created as psychedelic medicines come into our society. I believe a lot of that culture building is getting lost in the aboveground efforts. Reckoning with how we can acknowl-edge systems of oppression and how they impact our work with clients. The work happening at Alma is so important, but what are we doing as a broader community to create a safe, resilient culture around all of this? That feels like the work of the underground. And I think it's probably why there is a sense in the underground of feeling threatened by the fast-moving regulatory model that's happening.

RM: *Thank you for your courage and integrity in this work, and for pouring into me and so many others.*

Conclusion

Without shadow work we can never fully land or settle, because there will always be an element of avoidance in denial within ourselves and our communities.

Engaging with the shadow (and psychedelic work in general) asks us to expand our capacity to be present with many truths at once. It asks us to release ourselves from binary or reductionist thinking that separates things from one another. Again, we want to begin within ourselves and soften our relationships with our own shadows. But we can't stop there; the medicine for these times is developing the ability to hold our collective shadow and get to the root of it so we can heal it.

We can simultaneously hold that we are all parts of one unity consciousness, while recognizing that our lived realities harm some people while favoring others.

It is possible for experiences of union, oneness, and interconnectedness to activate us to live more justice-centered lives. But it's not a guarantee of psychedelic work; it requires us to integrate those experiences into meaningful action. In other words, the power of the transcendent experience lies in how it catalyzes us to move transformatively in our immediate spheres of influence.

The word *integrity* shares a root with the word *integrated;* it means to be intact. Whole medicine is possible when the shadow is acknowledged, honored, and invited into the conversation to find its healthy expression. Just as healing doesn't mean erasing what happened, much as we might prefer that, shadow work doesn't mean eradicating the rejected or unseen parts of ourselves. It means spending time developing compassion and curiosity for the shadow.

At the heart of healing is our relationship with the shadow. This chapter explored manifestations of shadow; other chapters explore resources for navigating the shadow, such as inner work, discernment, community, and accountability. In the coming chapters, we will explore the application of these principles in our medicine practice and work with clients.

CHAPTER 4

Discernment

People sometimes ask if I've ever had a "bad trip." I've been fortunate enough to consume substances in mostly supportive settings with people I trust, and even the ultra-challenging experiences I've had held teachings I'm now grateful for.

But there was this one time.

It was late summer, and the person I was dating kept a very well-stocked "pharmacy" of substances on hand. We'd spent most of the summer experimenting with different contexts and dosages; in fact, we rarely spent time together without consuming a psychedelic—which was otherwise rare for me. I had noticed a pattern of behavior in social settings where they would often "round up" and give people slightly more of a drug than they had asked for to make sure they "broke through." They seemed to have a high tolerance themself and a skewed idea of effective dosages for most people.

We took a laid-back camping trip alone to a beautiful lake in central Oregon. That night, I made a campfire and served dinner while they set up music and vibrant lights, and we took stock of our options for the evening.

"Let's try something out," they said.

They had already consumed a beer while we unpacked and proceeded to dose out a combination of GHB and ketamine. As I looked it over, it appeared to be more than a full dose of each, but I wasn't well versed in dosage. I voiced my hesitation and after a back and forth about "being on the same level," they slightly reduced the dose set for me. Their confident, nonchalant attitude made me second-guess my hesitations. We partook. A short while later, I realized that the amount I had consumed had launched me into an unmanageable high.

By then, the sun was setting and I felt a combination of loosening motor control and major dissociation coming on. I was rapidly losing access to my body, so I asked them to help me get some blankets. They did so and then wandered off to dance. I sat, bundled up in a camping chair, unable to move or speak, watching the campfire burn. My entire body was trembling uncontrollably. All of my senses separated out into distinct channels and I could only tune into one at a time. I sat there, immobilized, for about two hours.

I was convinced that I was going to be stuck in that chair until the fire went out and that I would freeze to death overnight. I had no idea where my travel mate had gone. I had a lengthy and unspoken conversation with the giant, magnificent fir trees and agreed that if this was my time to go, I had lived a good life. I cried silently. It felt palpably like a near-death experience (which I have since learned can happen with high doses of ketamine).

Finally, the effects began to ease and I was able to climb into their camper van and lie down. I woke up some time later to their crushing weight. They had climbed on top of me and promptly fallen asleep. I was still lacking access to my body, and lay there awake, laboring for each breath, again believing I might not survive the night. Finally, I shouted enough to wake them up, exclaiming, "Get off of me!" They rolled over and I was able to breathe.

At sunrise, I woke to the sound of birds. I could feel my hands and feet. I smiled. I went outside, weeping as the sun hit my face. I made a ceremonial fire and thanked my guardians for keeping me safe. My campmate stumbled into view just as the fire was turning to coals and asked if I wanted to take LSD after breakfast. I was baffled.

A few weeks later, I witnessed a similar situation at a festival where they gave a mutual friend a substance without checking what he had already consumed. This friend ended up in a psychedelic crisis that I had to help coordinate an entire care team to manage. I stopped dating this person shortly thereafter, and provided some difficult feedback about their reckless behavior. I learned the hard way that, while curiosity and experimentation hold value, they can lead to unsafe experiences if not balanced with consent, trust, and discernment.

Defining Discernment

Discernment—or wise, grounded judgment—is intricately linked with inner-work. The ability to discern is an outgrowth of compassionate, open-minded self-awareness. It requires slowing down, listening, asking, and reflecting on motives and beliefs. In many ways, our ability to cultivate discernment determines the success of our inner-work. When it comes to psychedelics, discernment extends beyond navigating individual consumption and whether or how to facilitate someone else's experience. It also includes intentionally deciding how we frame psychedelics within our spheres of influence, and what medicine communities we share our time and energy with.

The coming years will be rife with ever more opportunities and contexts to experience psychedelics. This is a result of rapidly shifting public opinion and policy shifts, as well as the economic forces that stand to turn a profit by increasing participation. Psychedelics are not right for everyone in all circumstances. And even when they are a good fit, more isn't always better. Additionally, becoming a psychedelic facilitator is certainly not a role right for everyone.

In our efforts to shift the public narrative about drug policy and nonordinary states of consciousness, it's important that we don't participate in dynamics that paint these complex substances as a panacea or minimize the potential risks. When that happens, we foster an inaccurate and counterproductive idea of the world of psychedelics, which can result in people being harmed and derail efforts to move beyond criminalization and prohibition.

Further, it's important to recognize that even with our best intentions and ideal set and setting, negative experiences and adverse events can (and do) happen with psychedelics. This can be due to a variety of factors, including misidentified or contaminated substances, interactions with existing medications, improper set and setting, underlying or undiagnosed medical or psychiatric conditions, and sometimes no clear explanation at all. On top of this, interpersonal harm such as misuse or abuse of power also sometimes occurs in psychedelic communities. By taking an honest look at these realities, we can make choices that minimize risk, maximize benefit, and enhance community safety.

If we want the promise of psychedelic medicine to be relevant for generations and fulfill its potential as an agent of collective healing, it's imperative that we develop the ability to discern when, how, and with whom to engage with psychedelics and consciousness-altering substances in ways that are suited for our unique contexts. These decisions will not only impact our immediate experiences, but the people around us, our communities, and the broader movement to normalize the exploration of altered states.

I spoke with Dr. Darron Smith to discuss the role of discernment for facilitators and clients.

Darron is an educator, researcher, writer, and professor based in Memphis, Tennessee. He received his PhD in the Department of Education, Culture, and Society at the University of Utah in 2010. Dr. Smith is a physician assistant with over fifteen years of experience in family and behavioral medicine. He is also an Army veteran, having served in Operation Iraqi Freedom. His practice is primarily within communities of color, including time spent on the Navajo reservation in southern Utah. With this mix of skills and training in sociology, he has a unique understanding of how social structures and institutions affect the health and well-being of individuals.

Within the psychedelic field, Dr. Smith has been recognized as a visionary leader by MAPS. He serves as a Board Member at the American Psychedelic Practitioners Association, a member of Chacruna Institute's Racial Equity and Access Committee, and was the first Director of Education at Alma Institute. Darron's insights are shared throughout this chapter.

When defining discernment, Darron says: "I see discernment as the wisdom people gain through experience. Living life, being knocked down, getting up again, and having the sense to listen to and be guided by one's mistakes. I see intuition as a flicker that comes and goes. Intuition can be fleeting. But discernment is a grounded skill that a person acquires over time."

Exploring Discernment

APPROACHES TO PSYCHEDELIC HEALING

In order for people to make sound decisions about where and how to engage with psychedelics, it's helpful to understand the nuances of different contexts. Generalizations about the way psychedelic practice should happen can be unhelpful; the field is too expansive for a singular approach. What's most important is that we each understand and abide by our unique scope of practice: that is, the style of work we are skilled, experienced, and prepared for. This can range from individual exploration, informal trip-sitting or group experiences with loved ones, informal communities of exploratory or spiritual practice, community-based guide work, nondirective psychedelic facilitation, and formal psychedelic-assisted therapies.

The psychedelic field has many forms of practice built on their own frameworks and theories regarding how healing and personal development happen. Healing is not always viewed as a unique emergent process driven by the participant. There are also top-down approaches where the participant is more of a recipient of a healing modality, the way one might receive a massage or acupuncture. In certain Indigenous contexts led by traditional medicine keepers, this can be well suited. In these cases, working with sacred plant medicines is treated as an intervention where the medicine person is the channel between realms. And in some cases, the participant does not actually consume any psychedelics at all—it is the medicine person who does.

Additionally, the methods employed by clinicians, therapists, and those with advanced or specialized training will rightfully differ from those used in peer-based practice. Those with extensive training in psychedelic-assisted therapies (PAT) will often take a more active role before, during, and after a psychedelic experience to help their patient or client prepare for, navigate, and interpret their experiences. These sessions are often held explicitly to address certain diagnoses or mental health challenges and adhere to tightly defined protocols.

A great deal of psychedelic use happens in less structured community contexts. For those new to psychedelics and existing outside of traditional Indigenous or clinical settings, a peer-supported approach rooted in the principles of harm-reduction is the natural entry point. One reason is that in most communities it's easier to find people experienced working with psychedelics than it is to get into a clinical trial or travel to another country to experience a traditional ceremony. The peer support or trip-sitting framework largely focuses on learning how to increase safety, maximize benefit, and get out of the way so natural processes can unfold. This method can be preferable because adding variables such as our own ideas, input, and perspectives to someone else's journey can often impede rather than support. In other words, the more we do during someone else's psychedelic experience, the more we risk interference. So we can start by stripping things back to the basics and learning to get comfortable actively doing less.

The nondirective approach stands in contrast to certain arenas in the field known today as psychedelic therapy. When we merge a top-down approach to healing with unexamined Western values and protocols, we risk imposing unacknowledged systems of hierarchy, consumerism, commodification, and appropriation into the medicine space and onto the people we are serving. Again, this is why it is so important to take the time to examine what we are bringing with us. Whatever our approach, the keys here are self-awareness and informed consent. It is crucial that facilitators and leaders of medicine groups be explicit with their philosophy, expectations, and agreements from the outset, and allow participants to ask questions and gain clarity before proceeding.

In spite of ongoing debate within the psychedelic field about how these powerful substances should enter society, we will never settle on just one homogenous way of practice. This is something to acknowledge and embrace. To illustrate, consider the wide variation in needs of people who are pregnant and giving birth. The spectrum of available care is correspondingly broad, because for some, giving birth at home with some basic supplies is perfectly safe. For others, monitoring and the presence of healthcare professionals are needed. Similarly, people seeking psychedelic experiences have widely different needs based on variables such as their mental health history, overall health and risk factors, and reasons for participation. It is our responsibility to ensure that this field is responsive to this wide spectrum of use and not overly prescriptive about the "best" approach.

EMBODIED AWARENESS

I asked Dr. Smith about his thoughts on the connection between somatics and discernment. "We need to be teaching and practicing discernment before people start working with clients," he said. He continued:

> This skill of discernment exists in the body and needs to be nurtured in new facilitators. Discernment can become more accessible if we help people tune into their gut, their nervous system, and their body. These

days, a lot of people haven't honed in on the ability to recognize what
their mind and body are telling them, what somatic cues and feelings
we are generating. Our behaviors conform to those sensations whether
they are conscious or not. In order to cultivate discernment we need to
first recognize somatic signals exist, then learn how to hear, process, and
honor them. This is ancient wisdom that we all hold (and science is now
catching up with ancient traditions). The range of people and experiences they have will be diverse. But we can all start in the body.

PSYCHEDELIC EVANGELISM

There is a common phase that occurs early in someone's relationship with psychedelic exploration. I call it "psychedelic evangelism." During this time, an
individual, having had a profound or transformative experience, attributes the
new insights and positive shifts in their life to the use of the substance. It's natural to conclude that if only everyone could take this substance or have this experience, they too could be healed, awakened, or transformed.

Engaging with an inexperienced community from this place of enthusiasm
comes with risks. Because there is still a lack of unbiased information and public
education around psychedelics, newcomers who hold little experience may be
rapidly propped up as relative experts within their friend circles, workplaces, or
communities. If this happens in tandem with an evangelism phase, what results
can be an oversight of risks, amplification of benefits, or reckless promotion of
unsupported use that leads to people getting hurt.

A great deal of understanding comes from years of practice. It also comes from
involvement within communities that have gleaned wisdom from direct experience and the collective sharing of core knowledge. As such, it's natural that folks
just starting out might not be totally aware of things like drug interactions, best
practices around set, setting, dose, and the psychological, physiological, or spiritual risks for certain groups—among other important factors to consider.

Additionally, there is a growing risk that substances sold as psychedelics
can be adulterated or entirely different substances than what they were sold
as. For this reason, it is best practice to *always* test your substances, even if you
trust the source and even if you are consuming in a casual social environment.
The risks of adverse events, overdoses, and even death continue to increase,
and testing is a simple practice that can be life-saving. There are kits readily
available online via groups such as DanceSafe and Test Your Poison. As people
who use substances or love people who do, we can do our part by normalizing
drug-checking and urging event organizers to make these services a mainstay
at their events.

Reaping benefits from a relationship with plant medicines and psychedelics requires more than access to substances. It's important to remember what we discussed in chapter 1, on Inner-Work: that our experiences of the world are not universal. There are many factors that contribute to having a positive experience with psychedelics, and just because you did, does not mean that your mother, neighbor, partner, or coworker will. Further, psychedelics don't automatically create prosocial changes in people. Consider the rise of New Age conspirituality (the melding of spirituality and conspiracy theories) and its connections with white supremacy, xenophobia, ableism, transphobia, and fascist ideology. This is not an issue that exists far away from this field; there is significant overlap and use of psychedelics and plant medicines in these subcultures, and harmful beliefs can proliferate with the suggestibility of altered states. That is to say, mass consumption is probably not the solution some imagine it to be.

SO YOU THINK YOU'RE A SHAMAN

There is another common phenomenon that occurs early in someone's journey with expanded states. That is the sense of calling. For many people, early journeys are marked as pivotal moments that shift the trajectory of their entire lives. This can be a positive thing when grounded in community and accountability. Many of the early insights and breakthroughs we have will be built upon over the coming years, through integration and the sacred practices that lie within ordinary life. With time, maturity, and context, the teachings of these substances weave their way organically into our paths and life decisions.

In other cases, a profound experience can also sometimes result in an inflation of one's ego and the sense of being "called" by the medicine. It's not an uncommon story, or a new one: a mentor with forty-plus years of experience in this culture explained to me that this is a long-standing pattern that precedes the current enthusiasm for psychedelics. Often, people will return from ceremonies abroad (sometimes facilitated by traditional medicine carriers and sometimes by Western-owned retreat centers) stating that they are selling their belongings, moving to another country, and pursuing the shamanic path. A sense of being unique and special, or the grand feeling of having received deep cosmic insights can be intoxicating. Opportunistic groups might even encourage these beliefs if there is something to be gained through your pursuit of a medicine path (such as retreats, collaborations, training courses, and so on). Remember that it can be very difficult to distinguish between our own inner narrator and the voice of the medicines. There is no real way to be sure, but time can be illuminating. Slowing down and practicing discernment are needed.

Because there is so much money to be made in this field, there is an increasingly varied ecosystem of psychedelic startups and service providers to choose from. With the added pressure of investment capital in certain business models, there is potential for conflict in priorities that, if not addressed, risk prioritization of scale and profit over quality of care. Find organizations and individuals aligned with your values, with a proven track record or vetted by people you trust—above- or underground.

Another question to consider is: why the urgency? If you are new to the work and feel called to serve medicine or be in a leadership role in any context, explore the possibility of giving yourself a year, or better yet, a few years, to be in a beginner's role and spend time under trusted mentorship. Working with medicine is a path of service, and it requires humility. It is better to do so while in the role of a student than in the role of a leader. Again, consider the "shadow why." Often, we'll find in ourselves a mix of sincere good intentions and less altruistic motives, such as an impulse toward self-advancement, a desire for notoriety, a craving to break free from the status quo and live an alternative lifestyle, or a hunger for purpose or meaning.

If the medicine is calling, there is truly no rush. There are time-honored reasons that traditional communities require many years of apprenticeship and humble service before serving medicine. There are ways to sustainably weave medicine work into your life without abandoning your current one.

Ultimately, radical shifts in one's life path are decisions each person must make on their own. However, the dynamics of power, privilege, entitlement, economics, colonialism, and maturity can all show up in the pursuit of serving medicine or working in this field. These all intersect when people—especially Westerners—become self-proclaimed healers or leap into leadership or business roles without honoring the customary rites of passage associated with such responsibilities. While these rites may be less obvious in grassroots medicine communities or legal psychedelic contexts, we know that healthy groups throughout society have clearly defined protocols and support the transfer of knowledge between generations. This is also true of psychedelic communities. In my experience, belonging within the broader psychedelic community is often connected with showing up with humility and consistency. We have the best outcomes when we put in the time, build and tend sincere, reciprocal relationships, and wait for our community to delegate us to roles of leadership.

There is room for a wide range of people in the psychedelic field, and I believe there is a general sense of openness to widening the circle. However, there are key principles and values that risk being lost or diluted when a cascade of folks move too rapidly from a learner's role into a leadership role. There is a great deal of history, nuance, and wisdom held in the existing communities of practice. To be a reliable representative of this field to the public, online, in the press, or in communities you are a part of, it's important to put in the time listening, learning, sitting quietly, and being of service. This not only reduces harm; it also builds trust among the existing network of incredible lineage keepers, guides, researchers, and policymakers who have dedicated many years to the work and taken great risks that benefit us today.

BENEFITS OF DEVELOPING DISCERNMENT

Finding a setting, facilitator, and context that is right for you can result in more transformative experiences. Every community and clinic has its own culture, ethos, and approach to the work. The experience you have will be informed by the person or group you choose to work with, and your level of comfort and rapport with them. Below are a few noteworthy benefits of making discernment part of your psychedelic path.

Connection with Inner Healer

When we move fast or ride on the confidence of others, it can be hard to connect with our own sacred knowledge. The path to finding a facilitator to work with can be medicinal in itself. It asks you to spend time reflecting, listening, and getting in touch with your own boundaries, needs, and desires. By increasing connection with your intuition, you strengthen the ability to hear and advocate for your deeper needs.

Reduced Risk

There are known facilitators and communities of practice who have a reputation for questionable ethics, patterns of harm, or lack of accountability. It can be hard for newcomers to recognize this, as many individuals and groups have adopted similar language. This makes it difficult to get a sense of someone's practices, approach, and the quality of care they bring to the work.

This is compounded by the fact that, in the United States and other places around the world, psychedelic facilitators and communities of practice exist in the shadows, making it difficult to know one group from another until you have spent time with them. Before working with anyone, take time to vet your practitioner, ask questions, and meet others in the community who know them. The Women's Visionary Congress published a list of twenty safety tips in 2014 that provides practical advice on minimizing risks when navigating ceremonial contexts at home and abroad.[1]

More Space for Integration

When we uncouple from the notion that more medicine is better, we begin to value the in-between periods, the liminal space between medicine experiences where altered states merge with daily life. By choosing not to engage in an endless loop of deep dives, we hold each experience with gravity. This means we will likely spend more time preparing for the experience, and we will be willing to lean into it fully, making the most of the time spent in an expanded state. We will commit to integration as a way of keeping the experience alive and honoring the gifts and insights given.

Conservation

Psychedelics don't just magically appear on our altars. Now we are collectively realizing that as a species, our lifestyles are out of balance with natural cycles. There is not an endless supply of psychedelic substances, and whether we are engaging with naturally occurring entheogens or lab-made compounds, each time we consume, we are using finite resources.

It is important, foundational even, to unlearn the consumer mindset in relation to psychedelic work. Engaging in a relationship or reciprocity often means slowing down and choosing to consume less, and less often to tread lightly on the earth. This practice is rooted in the Honorable Harvest, which is a teaching that permeates the worldviews of many original stewards of the land. We'll talk more about this in chapters 11 and 12, about History and Reciprocity.

Discernment in the Medicine Space

FOR JOURNEYERS

With more medicine circles and communities to choose from, it can be hard to know where to start. While the below items won't apply to everyone in all situations, here are some of the questions newcomers can consider as they navigate psychedelic services:

- What is the intention behind pursuing a psychedelic experience?
- What would a positive outcome look like to you?
- Have you spent time becoming aware of impulses toward urgency, escapism, or miracle cures that might impact your expectations of the experience?
- Are you prepared for things to get harder before you find lasting change or relief?

- Do you have a facilitator in mind already? Where are you planning to look?

- What qualities are important to find in a facilitator? What are your deal-breakers?

- Is it important that your facilitator has a matched identity or similar lived experience?

- What kind of training and orientation does the facilitator come from?

- What is the facilitator's belief system around how psychedelic healing works, and is it compatible with your own?

- In practical terms, what kind of experience are you prepared to have? Does it need to be local or abroad, and what kind of time and financial commitment are you prepared to make for prep, session, and integration?

Here are a few other key considerations for those who are navigating this rapidly changing scene.

SAFETY CANNOT BE GUARANTEED. Our lived experience impacts how we assess and experience risk. The safety of psychedelic spaces and journeys is not universally consistent, specifically for people who come from marginalized communities and have experienced direct and intergenerational trauma through many systems. Will the material that surfaces be met with understanding and compassion? Are there people present who share identifiers and can be in solidarity if issues do arise?

SPEND TIME WITH PEOPLE WHO ARE SKEPTICAL. This can be a healthy way of keeping early enthusiasm in check. Recognizing that a lot of mainstream belief about substance use has been shaped by the war on drugs can be useful to remember. However, this should not prevent us from being in community with people who are not supportive of our interest in psychedelics. It can prompt us to become clearer on our reasons and develop more nuanced attitudes around the work. In addition, there are plenty of people within psychedelic communities who maintain a healthy sense of skepticism. Spend time with them as well.

CARVE OUT TIME FOR QUIET AND REFLECTION. Develop a practice of self-care that allows you to be grounded, replenished, and connected to yourself. As discussed earlier, no one can track your preferences, needs, and boundaries as well as you can. Consider spending time with the questions above during your self-care rituals as a part of psychedelic preparation.

BE WILLING TO WAIT. In the process of your search, you may encounter signals or real-world barriers letting you know that it is not the right time to pursue a big experience. Consider the benefits of spending time in preparation and explore what other supportive modalities could be a part of a more gradual healing process. Sometimes receiving a "no" or "not now" can be a blessing in disguise.

CONNECT WITH COMMUNITY. Psychedelic societies, conferences, forums, and trusted news sources can all help you form a more informed outlook so you can navigate the space with clarity. Just be sure to not only surround yourself with psychedelic enthusiasts, as this can create a skewed outlook via psychedelic evangelism. Look for people who seem to be trusted elders and have a grounded outlook on the benefits and limitations of psychedelics.

FOR FACILITATORS

Here are a few general rules for facilitators working with clients:

1. Do your learning. Work to understand the ways risks are different for people based on their health history, social location, and unique situation. Encourage them to spend time getting in touch with their own intuition and support their agency in making the decision of whom to work with.

2. Tell the truth. Answer direct questions with direct answers. Better yet, provide them with an externally provided list of questions, such as "Questions to Discuss with a Prospective Psychedelic Facilitator" by Fireside Project. This way people can make decisions from a fully informed place, which reduces risk and is just the right thing to do.

3. Get comfortable with saying "I don't know," and get advice or guidance from elders and mentors. Maintain a learner's attitude, and never overstate your experience or qualifications.

Considerations for people interested in entering into facilitation work:

SCOPE OF PRACTICE CAN BE FLUID BASED ON SETTING. Facilitators need to be able to discern what kind of support is appropriate in each context, especially when trained in a variety of modalities. For example, there may be facilitators shifting from informal harm-reduction settings into more structured facilitation work, or facilitators moving from underground facilitation into psychedelic-assisted therapies. It is important to be aware of how the goals, protocols, and boundaries of psychedelic work can differ from one context to another.

In my experience, there is a common adage within regulated access models that encourage professionals to "leave their credentials at the door," in favor of the nondirective approach to psychedelic work. In other words, this suggests that someone with existing credentials (e.g., a therapist or nurse) should only operate within the scope of a nondirective facilitator while providing psychedelic care. However, it is impossible to fully disengage from existing skill sets, and they can be beneficial. In addition, licensure under various regulatory boards might require a person such as a trained medical professional to intervene in medical emergencies, while this behavior would be inappropriate for a facilitator without such credentials.

People who come to you might subconsciously expect you to be their therapist, pharmacist, and doctor all at once. Be extremely clear and up front about your training, skills, and approach to the work, and voice any concerns that you might not be the best fit.

WE ALL HAVE BLIND SPOTS. Commit to ongoing relationships with elders and community. We each need peer consultation and mentorship, no matter how many years we have been practicing personally or holding space for others. While we can gain wisdom and insight through practice, we are never done healing or learning. Through learning, we become aware of our own humanity and vulnerability. We need each other.

When engaging with an elder or mentor, reflect on what reciprocity might look like. Intergenerational learning is one of the most human traditions we have. It would be a missed opportunity to not engage with the many people in this field who have decades and lifetimes of experience working with medicine in a variety of contexts.[2] How can you give back to the person who is imparting their support, guidance, and wisdom to you? While it can be hugely rewarding to have your apprenticeship honored and recognized, we can go further to really make mentoring the next generation a rewarding experience for those who have walked the medicine paths before us.

DON'T RUSH THE PREPARATION. Regardless of the context you are working in, screening and intake are some of the most important predictors of how beneficial a session will be. Establish a consistent system you can abide by repeatedly. What happens during intake is critically important to what happens on the journey day. Make a list of red-, yellow-, and green-light clients based on your levels of training, expertise, comfort, and personal triggers/boundaries.

COLLABORATE. If you are a grassroots provider, it is ideal to find a trusted therapist, a psychedelic-savvy pharmacist, and/or a medically trained professional in your inner circle for consultation. These are people you can call on in the process of screening to gain clarity on whether someone is the right fit to work with you. Mental health history and drug interactions should be taken seriously. It is not an immediate red flag to work with people who have more complex health situations; however, an untrained individual—even with good intentions—might overlook risk factors that a medical or mental health professional can catch.

BE CLEAR ABOUT RISKS. Spend time looking closely at the research and listening to stories of less optimal experiences. Volunteer in a harm-reduction context like the Zendo Project. Do what you need to have a sober outlook on this work, and convey a balanced attitude. Discuss and manage expectations for your clients. In this process you'll come to understand what they are looking for and how fixed or flexible their expectations are. This can help you discern whether you are the right person to work with them.

PRACTICE THE GUT CHECK. Trust goes both ways. You should be able to sense the trust of your client, and you should hold trust in their intentions, capacity, and honesty. If this healing alliance isn't or can't be established, take some time on your own to explore why that might be. A poor facilitator-client match is a recipe for negative outcomes. If you do not feel comfortable working with someone, it is far better to refer them to someone else than to move forward.

In that vein, be sure you have a referral network of skilled, trusted facilitators who hold different skill sets or modalities than you. If, upon reflection, you do not believe psychedelic work is right for someone who wants to work with you, be clear on your reasons. Without making judgments about their mental health, personality, or readiness for the work, communicate this. It can be enough to compassionately share the core reasons you can't move forward and that your personal and professional boundaries don't allow you to work with them. Refer when you can or recommend alternatives to psychedelic work, being sure not to diagnose or prescribe in any fashion outside of your scope of practice.

TRAINING IS IMPORTANT. Dr. Smith shared the following:

> The training programs have a real responsibility here. When we're bringing people into programs, we need to assess whether that facilitator has been doing their inner-work. That's where the faculty member who is doing the initial interview needs to be able to really listen to a person's soul. We need references from people who have known them for a long time. We need to take the time to get a good sense of who people are, and only certify or graduate people who we have the utmost confidence in. People who will exercise discernment and embrace mentorship.

PUBLIC EDUCATION AND TRUTH TELLING: FOR THE FIELD-BUILDERS

Psychedelic field-builders have unique responsibilities around discernment. The future health of our communities depends on us practicing discernment in all of the above areas, as well as in driving policy change and public education.

The best thing we can do is take a balanced approach and embrace a narrative grounded in facts. It's not just about managing the narrative, even though we do at times need to be strategic because we are dealing with stigmatized substances and widespread misinformation. We also need to tell the truth about the risks, potential benefits, adverse events, and limitations of these substances. Not just in the public forum, but in policy efforts, donor/investor meetings, fact-based journalism, accurate reporting, and awareness campaigns. We need to set aside the motives of PR and profitability, in favor of public safety. This means finding the balance between highlighting the legacy of safe community and ceremonial use, and telling the truth about risks. Doing so can help manage expectations, prevent backlash and opposition, and drive support for risk reduction practices and safety nets.

Honing our ability to a) hear our inner voice and b) honor the direction of that intelligence shapes the way we make decisions in everyday life. We will also learn to recognize and value this in other people. When we begin collectively exercising discernment, it can feed into the culture of an organization. Group decision-making processes become more collaborative when grounded in a willingness to slow down and gain clarity.

For example, at Alma Institute, we have often been in a position of receiving outside pressures to move faster, scale bigger, and expand more broadly. We are working to create a culture of slowing down, somatic awareness, and embracing shared decision-making so we can stay in line with our values and stated goals, and course-correct when we begin to get derailed. I rarely regret slowing down. It gives us a chance to find our center, share understanding, and explore possible next steps.

In Conversation with Alissa Bazinet, PhD

Alissa Bazinet is a licensed clinical psychologist, research scientist, and psychedelic therapist in Portland, Oregon. She is the cofounder of Sequoia Center, a nonprofit community clinic offering affordable and accessible psychedelic services, including ketamine-assisted psychotherapy and psychedelic integration counseling. As a member of the Oregon Psilocybin Advisory Board's training subcommittee, she contributed to the development of initial rules and regulations for state-sanctioned psilocybin facilitator training programs. She is also a longtime volunteer for psyche-delic peer support organizations at music festivals and events. She is passionate about harm-reduction, informed consent, and the ethical provision of psychedelic services.

RM: *When I say the word* discernment, *what comes to mind for you?*

AB: In the context of psychedelic services, *discernment* means "meeting each individual where they are." Really doing our best as providers to understand what considerations are needed in order for them to have a positive outcome. So, rather than thinking in terms of whether someone is an "appropriate candidate" for services, whether we should screen them in or out, it's more a question of what is needed for this person in this particular situation to have an experience that is beneficial and not harmful.

RM: *When it comes to beginner education, do you see any examples of public education that you think are working well?*

AB: I feel like we're in the very beginning stages of actually launching some of those ideas for public education. So far, it seems like Fireside Project and the surrounding efforts to build awareness of the hotline have been really effective. It's one-on-one peer support and integration. With this format, Fireside is able to meet the needs of a lot of different kinds of people and contexts, whereas psychedelic societies and integration circles can sometimes have a more homogenous attendee base. We can now send ketamine clients to Fireside for additional support. They've had really positive experiences.

At Sequoia, we've been dreaming up an education campaign for various types of healthcare providers and settings. We'd like to roll out training "within the system" at community mental health clinics, hospitals, emergency rooms, and local primary care offices. As of now, the majority of healthcare providers are misinformed. And that's where a lot of people who may not have familiarity or comfort with psychedelics or psychedelic culture are going to ask questions. Because, for example, they saw a campaign ad on TV that said psilocybin can treat anxiety and depression. So they're going to ask their primary care provider about that.

This kind of education needs to come from those of us who are bridges between psychedelic communities and healthcare structures and systems. We don't want an entire network of providers who are ill-equipped when their patients come with questions.

RM: *For those of us who end up providing services, what do we need to do in order to make space for people who are dealing with more complex health situations?*

AB: I think it will come down to coordination with multiple types of care providers. We already see this within existing healthcare structures and in the community too. For example, I think the Veterans Affairs hospital system does a really great job with the interdisciplinary care model. A veteran's treatment team often includes their psychiatrist, psychologist, or social worker; as well as peer support individuals who are also veterans and have lived through similar situations. That peer support person provides solidarity and helps the veteran get the appointments they need and find the appropriate services.

Within states that are legalizing psychedelic access, we need to establish a similar model. I, as a clinical provider, need to be able to work with care providers who work in a community-based context. And hopefully, there can be reciprocity and relationship there.

Conclusion

As psychedelics become mainstream, we have an opportunity to model discernment and set the tone of grounded, balanced decision-making for the general public. This creates a culture of agency and responsibility. When we acknowledge that there *are* risks with this work and that negative events *do* sometimes happen, we accomplish a few things. First, we create space for people to make informed decisions about whether to participate. Second, we can help prevent occasional negative events from derailing the public narrative or feeding into stigma about these substances. Third, we create safety plans that can help address and mitigate risks, helping improve outcomes over time.

Developing discernment happens on the individual and the community/movement level. Like most of the pillars of practice, it is fractal. We cultivate these skills and practices in our individual lives, and we find others who are doing the same. Then we are able to organize, form coalitions, and make bigger, weightier decisions collectively that are still grounded in our hearts, bodies, and integrity. In some ways, collective decision-making can be more conducive to discernment because we have the benefit of checks and balances through partnering with one another; no one person's blind spot or growth edge has enough sway to derail a major decision. The key is to surround ourselves with people who are also doing their inner-work, willing to slow down, and able to listen not only to themselves but to one another.

Discernment is foundational to good decision-making, but it is only one part of it. Discernment comes from awareness, but it requires meaningful action to fulfill its potential.

CHAPTER 5

Community

When I was a child, my mother would send me next door to borrow an egg or a cup of flour from the neighbors. This was part of the social order and an unspoken agreement of the times. It said: We hold one another up. My thriving and safety are tied up in yours. Your pain is my pain. This is an intimacy I don't see often these days. In an age of hyper-connectivity, it's easier to pay for a stranger to deliver eggs to your doorstep via an app than to interact with someone whose whole home and life exist just a few yards away from your own.

Growing up in the Church, I found that one of its saving graces was the strength of a committed community. These families did not just worship and pray together; they raised children, navigated illness and loss, celebrated rites of passage, supported during crises, and shared in the less remarkable but altogether worthwhile moments of life. Bonded by shared beliefs, the church community fostered a deep sense of belonging. As a child, I was rescued from drowning in a pond by a close friend, only to later learn that her father had saved my mother from drowning in a lake when they were teenagers. I insistently joked that our future children only swim together.

Since I left religious institutions, it's been harder to find that level of intact community. During the awkward years after Bible college, there was one place I always felt myself: the garden. I was a member of several land projects during that period that gave me a grounding and sense of self via community.

First, I joined a farm cooperative run by a family at the church. They were the first people who taught me the basics of growing food. The commitment required that we chip in some funds at the beginning of the season and participate in communal work days: in exchange, we were invited to come harvest crops as they became ripe and gather for farm parties and seasonal celebrations. I grew wildflowers for my wedding. We participated in life-death cycles. We hand-fed cows and sheep. They grew up, and through tears, I bore witness to their inevitable slaughter and participated in meat-packing days that felt more like a ceremony than sustenance.

Later, I joined the board of directors at a local farmers market. The weekend rituals of roaming the aisles became a new version of church. I became close friends with many of the farmers, lingering at their booths, sewing clothes for their babies, and receiving heirloom seeds they'd saved like treasures at the end of the season. I noticed the simple comfort of being bonded by land and food, beyond dogma and across differences.

Years later, through psychedelic explorations, I found a close inner circle with whom I wanted to share more of life. They were a group I trusted enough to embark on adventures through drug-induced alternate dimensions at festivals. Yet, they were grounded enough to share meals and help one another through life's changes. In my heart, I wanted to bridge the gap between friendship and family. My partner and I began hosting weekly dinners and we all began to dream of forming a village.

When a core friend inherited a large property outside of the city, we were thrilled. They asked me if I would join them in creating a land-based intentional community. In my eagerness, I jumped at the opportunity and started to organize group efforts to make it a reality. But I was moving out of pace with my friends, and I was met with resistance. I couldn't see the ways I was projecting my hunger for a secure community onto the group and derailing the efforts in the process. The project unraveled. The group cooled off, not because of any major rupture, but because we didn't have the language or skills to navigate difficulties and shifts within our relationship.

This experience impacted the way I approach community. I've learned that a community is only as strong as its ability to hold conflict and foster repair. I've learned that affection isn't enough to create lasting bonds; we need commitment, shared agreements, pacing, and enough softness to bend and not break.

Defining Community

The way we define community is shaped by the beliefs we hold about the world and our place in it. Community is everyone you are connected with. This connection can come from geographical proximity, shared interests, values, and identities. Our lives do not and cannot exist in isolation. When partaking in psychedelics, we often receive lessons from the natural world: among the most common is that we are all interconnected in a web of life. No matter how disconnected modern humans have become from this notion, it is a veritable fact. Psychedelic practice does not stop at personal healing and growth; beyond that lies the potential to transform our homes, lives, and communities. Fortunately, there are tools and resources that enable us to create more resilient communities. It is slow and relational work, but I believe it's work that we can't afford *not* to do.

Exploring Community

Before sharing the following reflections, I want to acknowledge four women mentors who have shaped my beliefs about what community means, both within and beyond the psychedelic space: Hanifa Nayo Washington, Diana Quinn, Claudia Cuentas, and Annie Oak. Women and gender-expansive people have been at the heart of community care throughout human history, and continue to hold essential wisdom, power, and cultural practices. When we lift women up with integrity and support their leadership, we build communities that are strong, resilient, and beautiful. These women are just a few of the leaders I believe we should be looking at, to guide us in building and shaping the psychedelic fields in the coming years.

AN EPIDEMIC OF LONELINESS

We need each other. Being together is as ancient as history itself. Intact communities of Indigenous people never forgot this very basic truth. The importance of communion—togetherness—is not just a nice idea. It is essential to our well-being and survival. Community is where we come together to address the problems of our time. Community is an antidote to authoritarianism. It is the alternative to policing and surveillance culture. It is where we are reminded of who we are and what we're capable of. It is family; it is home.

But we are a rapidly disconnecting species. The United States, and Western culture at large, is hyper-individualistic. It has never been so easy for us to avoid interacting with or relying on one another. We can choose to scan our own groceries, have contactless delivery for almost anything, text our loved ones rather than call, and form entire "social" networks with people we might never meet. We even have sex robots and VR systems to liberate us from true human intimacy. This is a global experiment in disconnection.

The US Surgeon General has classified this phenomenon as an "epidemic of loneliness." An abundance of strong scientific research clearly demonstrates that loneliness and isolation contribute to chronic stress, and chronic stress in turn contributes to countless other diseases. One prominent researcher, Steve Cole, PhD, found that loneliness can alter the behavior of immune cells by upregulating inflammatory gene expression. "Loneliness acts as a fertilizer for other diseases," Dr. Cole said. "The biology of loneliness can accelerate the buildup of plaque in arteries, help cancer cells grow and spread, and promote inflammation in the brain leading to Alzheimer's disease. Loneliness promotes several different types of wear and tear on the body."[1]

HEALING SPACES

Community is not just a backdrop where our lives play out. It is our place of origin and the place we return to. We each exist because our community made us. The communities of ancestors, family members, lands, plants, animals, traditions, and lifeways. Community is bound up with culture, with the visible and invisible tapestries that make up human life. For this reason, access to community can also be the site of profound healing. Being embraced and welcomed into a collective can be a corrective, reparative experience for those who have experienced being on the outside.

Many of our wounds are not just familial. They can also be connected to dysfunctional, harmful, or nonexistent communities. For many, the first experiences of community happen in the family, the block, school, or church. Communities naturally form wherever we exist, grow, and survive. Just as in family lines, communities can carry collective trauma that becomes culture. These, too, are places that hold opportunities for healing and transformation. But healing community begins within ourselves.

Community can be weaponized. All too often, predatory actors, forces, and impulses take advantage of our fundamental need for belonging. For me, having grown up in the Christian Church, "You're going to hell" represented the ultimate exiling. It meant being eternally cut off from God, as well as community. That is how important community is—that the worst punishment the creators of a world religion could think of was to strip someone of it. Some communities do have policies of expelling people, and clearly communicate the circumstances under which this might occur: usually when harm occurs for group safety. There are ways to compassionately stop people from doing harm while honoring the humanity of all involved. Unfortunately, more often in society, exiling is a reactionary and violent tactic—such as in the criminal legal system.

Community is the soil where humans and other living beings grow. Healthy community provides fertile nourishment, while isolation leads to famine. When people are starved of healthy connections, they fail to thrive. We can't have a serious conversation about healing without putting community at the center.

CHOSEN FAMILY

Let's get one thing straight: community is not all sunshine, rainbows, and barbecues. It is often messy. One of humanity's most important evolutionary successes has been learning how to be with one another through significant differences. But it gets harder when we've fallen out of practice—if we were ever fortunate enough to experience a functional community to begin with. By their very nature, unfettered capitalistic values are antithetical to our social fabric. The late-stage capitalist narrative manufactures scarcity: its nearly exclusive focus on competition, and total disregard for collaboration—which is at least as strong an evolutionary force as competition—cuts us off from one another to deadly ends. This narrative says there is not enough for everyone, so we must compete to satisfy our basic needs. We must climb on one another to fulfill our ultimate purpose: winning at all costs. These are lies, but we are afraid, so we act like they are true.

In light of this, we can form microcosms of the societies we would like to live in. We can set up environments where we actively disrupt ideas of scarcity and competition and form collective agreements that prompt us to trust one another. We can experience the plenty that is possible when we gather, celebrate culture, and build collective power. Groups who have shared experiences of oppression know something about the deep community that folks in dominant culture rarely experience fully. Collaborative and caring bonds are often forged on the margins.

ACROSS AFFINITY AND GEOGRAPHY

What makes a healthy community? There's so much to unpack there. But at a glance, here are a few things to consider:

- A shared identifier, goal, interest, or locale that unifies the community
- Diversity of lived experiences
- Shared power and collective decision-making processes
- The ability to shift and evolve in response to changing needs
- The ability to embrace disagreement and conflict as generative and natural processes
- The capacity for rupture and repair
- Clear parameters for expulsion applied fairly across the community
- The willingness to support the agency and unique thought of individual members
- The promotion of prosocial behaviors such as sharing of resources
- Willingness to care for those with differing needs
- Mutual accountability and systems for addressing harm when it occurs

It is aspirational to find ways to repair relationships when ruptures happen. The throwaway culture is one that ultimately will have to change if we are going to course-correct; at the same time, a lack of consequences or actionable responses to violence can dissolve communities as well. Reactionary punishment and impunity are both vulnerabilities that need to be addressed. We'll talk more about this in chapter 10, on Accountability.

There is value in many forms of community. Organized, structured communities are easier to find, provide clearer containers for newcomers, can be built with lasting power, set their own rules, and grow toward shared goals. They can also provide models for surrounding communities. On the other hand, communities that function as decentralized networks, such as mutual aid networks and interest or affinity-based groups that are connected digitally, have the ability to be more agile and responsive to their environment. They create less of a distinction between in and out and thus have a lower barrier to access.

A coalition is a community of communities. This is where the fractal nature of psychedelic work really comes into focus. Just as individuals participate in communities, there are many organizations that participate in larger communities as coalitions that make up what we call the psychedelic ecosystem. Many of the same dynamics and challenges we face in single communities apply here and are amplified. Just as with individuals in a community, a coalition is made stronger by the diversity of its members. Diversity leads to resilience. None of us knows everything, and together we know a lot. This is multiplied when we embrace the value of elders in our communities and support the sharing of wisdom across generations.

For those working in the psychedelic field, it is worth slowing down and considering whether your project needs to be a structured, organized community or whether you can participate in a decentralized network. It depends on the goals. It is wise to be cautious of the impulse to create another "thing." Sometimes there is a need, and other times this can pull resources (public energy, funding, volunteers, attention, labor) from existing groups that could benefit from your involvement.

Community in the Medicine Space
FOR JOURNEYERS

It is so valuable to have a welcoming, understanding place to process your psychedelic experiences. However, it might not be necessary or even helpful to lean on a psychedelic-specific group for this. Consider who is already in your life, whom you share trust, openness, and support with. Embrace the value of these existing communities. Learn the warning signs of a cult or a community with cult-like tendencies. Turn to psychedelic circles for support specific to medicine work, but be careful not to discard or deprioritize your other webs of relationships in the process.

Psychedelic communities can be beautiful places of understanding and integration. However, they also risk becoming echo chambers run by enthusiasts or even fanatics that can grow increasingly disconnected from the rest of the world. These communities risk taking on cult dynamics.

Signs of Cult Dynamics

1. Authority of a charismatic leader, guru, or medicine person
2. Us versus them/insider–outsider belief system where the group/leader holds the truth

3. Double standards—members abide by one set of standards, but leaders are above those rules

4. Suppression of doubts or critical thinking

5. Use of defense-weakening practices such as prayer, meditation, chanting, and altered states of consciousness

6. Delegitimizing of past members and critics

7. Encouraging disengagement from outside community

8. Abuse of power by leaders, often in the realms of sex, money, or personal gain

9. Lack of transparency around financial gain, governance, or past scandals

10. Inner circles, secret councils, or veiled operations that encourage mystery and intrigue

11. Preoccupation with keeping or gaining members, threats of punishment for speaking out

Healthy Psychedelic Communities

1. Enable their participants to come and go freely

2. Encourage participation in other communities

3. Engage and collaborate with local groups not involved with psychedelics

4. Foster an environment of sincerity where belonging is not contingent on being homogenous with other members

5. Are committed to improving and evolving

6. Share key decisions and responsibilities among a few people rather than a single individual

7. Solicit and meaningfully respond to feedback

8. Establish and uphold systems for accountability, applied consistently regardless of position

9. Are transparent and honest with their members about their leadership, power, and decision-making structures

FOR FACILITATORS

Networks of peer support provide contexts for all of us to grow, learn, improve, heal, and prevent harm. Community is a crucial component of healing and support for clients. Daily life is where teachings and insights become habits. Facilitators should reinforce the importance of community for our clients and create our medicine practices with support systems and integration networks.

People often want to start their own projects during their psychedelic evangelism phase. It's like the honeymoon phase of psychedelics. We want all we do between waking and sleeping to be about psychedelics. It's possible this could be a misplaced or misguided expression of the need to integrate.

When this happens, instead of taking the insights and healing imparted by the medicine and weaving it into our lives' context, we see people changing their identities, habits, social circles, and even ideals in order to feel closer to the psychedelic experience. This is concerning for a couple of reasons: first, it can have a negative impact on people who aren't part of the psychedelic subculture. They can feel pushed out or cast aside, and this can feed into the dynamic where psychedelic communities become actual or perceived cults, drawing loved ones away from the community.

Instead of inviting members of the public into a psychedelic community to assimilate, groups of psychedelic practice can adapt to reflect their memberships and promote diversity of thought, lifestyle, and demographics. They can find ways to integrate with the local community that do not rely on altered states, such as art, music, movement, meditation, and spiritual practice. This is important for the health and lasting power of organizations. We each can play a part in shaping the culture of our individual networks, which will ultimately coalesce in the coming years to create a composite image of this moment in psychedelic history. It will shape public perception and press coverage, which can influence public policy and public support. It matters how we organize ourselves in this emerging field.

In Conversation with Victor Cabral

I had the joy of working with Victor in 2021 as part of a JEDI (Justice, Equity, Diversity, and Inclusion) committee in the psychedelic field. I was struck by his groundedness, wisdom, and vision for community healing. In the time I have known him, I have seen him blossom into what I believe will be one of the leading voices in the next generation of psychedelic stewardship.

Victor Cabral is a collaborative leader committed to making an impact on historical inequities in his community and beyond. He is a licensed social worker and practicing psychotherapist in Pennsylvania with training in Internal Family Systems and psychedelic-assisted therapy. At the time of this interview, Victor served as the Director of Policy and Regulatory Affairs for Fluence Training. He is listed on Students for Sensible Drug Policy's (SSDP) list of "40 Under 40 Outstanding BIPOC

Leaders in Drug Policy in the United States" for his work in psychedelic policy, and received the 2022 Emerging Social Work Leader Award from the National Association of Social Workers (NASW).

RM: *What does community mean to you?*

VC: I experience community as the people who are closest to the experiences that I've had, who can understand and empathize with my life, and vice versa. Through this, we find this space where we can support one another through those connections. And so I think community is this intangible thing—like this energy field where people feel safe with one another, where people understand and care for one another, and recognize the ways we are all interconnected. In community, people are working for the larger good of that collective energy, rather than just for themselves.

I believe we each have our own parts to heal and roles to play within this larger system. And then when we come together, the whole is greater than the sum of its parts. And that's a beautiful thing to be part of. That's healing in itself.

RM: *Can you describe what that means when we talk about intergenerational healing?*

VC: In my journey, there was this initial awakening to life. Coming to see more clearly all the things that I had been through, all the things that had happened to me and the people around me. And as I worked through those things, I naturally started to dig deeper and deeper. I started to ask: "Where did this come from?"

When we do that, we start to trace patterns back over generations and see how certain traumas were handed down. For me, intergenerational healing means looking beyond my individual experience in this lifetime and starting to see how that trauma came from somewhere before me, in my lineage.

At first, waking up to the realities and recognizing that what happened is not your fault can bring up a lot of anger. You might think: I was let down. This shouldn't have happened. And that anger has its place. But we can't stay there forever. Ultimately, we can move beyond that into this place of compassion.

As I did that work of untangling the history, I think that's how the healing started to happen. I started to hold the same understanding and compassion for my ancestors, my mother, and my father, that I was holding for myself. I recognized that the things that happened to me weren't my fault. The things that happened to my parents and ancestors weren't their fault, either.

The next step after that was, "How do I take this knowledge and this wisdom that I've received, apply it to my life, and begin to heal? How do I break free from this cycle?" I had this stage where I was trying to heal all of my family's drama. I realized really quickly that this was adding to my distress, trying to fix and heal everyone else.

But what is within my sphere of influence is myself and how I raise my daughters. So I began thinking about how I can lead a different path for them.

Psilocybin helped me pause and see what was happening and make a change.

RM: *How has your experience been in your community with people who have different viewpoints or experiences?*

VC: That's one of the things that I've learned from dear friends of mine who are wisdom holders and medicine holders. They always used to tell me, "You don't push anyone into this work." And that's hard to wrap your head around when you first start to heal because you want everyone else to heal. I've been doing medicine work for such a long time, and even still, I have these really difficult moments of knowing more about who I am and yet having to do more work. Those moments really make me reflect on what an individual path this is. You have to choose it for yourself.

RM: *How would you imagine these psychedelic or plant medicines weaving with other forms of public health work, activism, and other communities?*

VC: The psychedelic field is still in a bubble and it has the potential to bring out the darkest nature of who we are as well—the ego, greed, and misuse of power. I think what keeps us from getting lost in the shadow side of psychedelics is our tethering to community. So when I speak or participate at a conference, I come home and my community humbles me and reminds me where I come from and why I am doing all of this.

So when I think about how this can impact society, I think about what it can look like for the small city that I'm from. It has 100,000 people. What if all our community leaders did healing work, and what if all our citizens had access to that healing work? There's an empowerment that builds around that, which allows those communities to mobilize and impacts social justice, equity, public health, and all of these other sectors.

That way we are mobilizing from a place of love. A place of soul and understanding our interconnectedness. And I think that's so much more impactful. Movements are often reactions to injustice and righteous anger. They're often pitted against each other over resources. Then it's easy for those movements to fall apart. One community gets resources and the other one doesn't.

When you're working with these medicines, they're reminding us of the important elements. Why are we here? What is our relationship to each other? What is our guiding direction? If it's love and soul and community, I think that just changes the fabric of how we engage with every aspect of our society.

In Conversation with Annie Oak

Annie Oak is a rare presence in the psychedelic ecosystem. She has witnessed and participated in its ongoing evolution for over four decades, and remains a leading and influential figure, across subcultures, in its current iteration. Annie is someone who embodies her values, uplifts those around her, and holds power in a way I deeply admire. She's also as fun as she is fierce. I want to be like Annie when I grow up.

Ann Harrison is a journalist based in San Francisco. She has covered business, science, and politics for numerous news organizations including Wired News, Fast Company, Agence France-Presse, and several National Public Radio member stations. After working for several years as a technology reporter, Ann began writing about gray market economies. In 2020, Ann cofounded Lucid News, where she presently serves as managing editor. She has an MS in science reporting from the Columbia University School of Journalism. In 2007, Ann began cocreating companies and organizations under the name Annie Oak. She founded the Women's Visionary Congress and cofounded its parent organization, the Women's Visionary Council, the first nonprofit for psychedelic women. Recognizing the need to provide a quiet, comfortable space at music festivals, Ann created the Full Circle Tea House as a collaborative community art project. Ann is also the cofounder of Take 3 Presents, a San Francisco-based event production company that produces immersive art experiences. A longtime public health activist, Ann develops risk-reduction strategies for event organizers. She is a resident of San Francisco's Haight-Ashbury neighborhood.

With a seasoned history of active involvement in psychedelic communities, Annie has taught me a great deal about community ethics, accountability, and the importance of lifting up elders and wisdom keepers. There is nothing so humbling as when an esteemed role model reaches out and says, "I want to help you," and that is what Annie has done for me.

RM: *Can you share a bit about yourself and how you came to this work?*

AO: I think it's important to talk a little bit about my own background because we all bring our own perspectives and biases to our work. I have a different perspective than others would. I'm sixty-one years old and I've been a member of different psychedelic communities since the 1970s. I was sometimes a very joyous participant in those communities. Certainly, my interactions with psychedelics have brought me healing, personal insight, joy, and connection with the communities I'm part of.

Sometimes, those experiences have been challenging for me, both my engagement with psychedelic compounds and also things that have happened to me within those communities. I have, like many, many people, been assaulted, abused, coerced, harassed, and all of that. That's not specific to psychedelic communities; that, unfortunately, is often part of the world we live in. But I think it can be more challenging when that happens within psychedelic communities, because we are by definition, communities of outlaws. We're drug users. We're people who seek to expand our consciousness in different ways. We're activists and healers. Anybody who is a certain age is, by definition, an outlaw if they were involved with psychedelics. We like to say that.

So, within communities where you're already engaging in activities that are outside the law, how do you hold people accountable and support harm-reduction within those communities? Because, if something happens to you at a festival where psychedelics were used, you might be more hesitant to reach out to law enforcement, or other outside systems of justice or accountability, because you don't want to be seen as a traitor, betraying your community, or bringing the eyes of the law on to you. We know that all people have a right to expand their consciousness without being coerced and abused and manipulated and assaulted. That's a human right.

RM: *We need to name that we all are capable of harm and need to be doing our inner-work and looking for channels for repair, while also cautioning the broader community about red flags, because people could get really hurt.*

AO: Discernment is very, very important. I believe we're having a kind of "hearts and flowers" moment with psychedelics right now. There are a lot of people who are coming to these experiences and these compounds with fresh eyes and open hearts. And that's so essential, and so needed at this moment in time. And yet, at the same time, there's a certain naivete that comes with that.

I think it's very important for people to understand that psychedelics put people in a very suggestible and flexible frame of mind. That mindset is essential for healing, working through trauma, being ourselves, and connecting to the earth and our community. But it can also be manipulated and abused by people who are predators. They exist within psychedelic communities as therapists, shamans, and facilitators. And because there are opportunities to harm and manipulate people, it attracts those kinds of predators and we need to understand that. Be discerning, do your due diligence, and be mindful of red flags.

RM: *I wonder how it has been for you, as someone who has been a part of this space for forty-plus years? For most of that time, the psychedelic business was not the phenomenon it is now; money wasn't the driving force that it's become in the last ten or so years. How do you experience this stark shift toward commodification?*

AO: It's been interesting to watch. Those of us who are paying attention are not surprised to see us at this present moment. A lot of effort, thoughtful activism, and research by well-intentioned people—and also a great deal of money—has gone into making people aware of the strong potential that psychedelic compounds have for healing. The resulting explosion of therapies, studies, companies, retreat centers, and legislation is inevitable. It's the result of years and years of dedicated activism from people who put everything on the line for this. They took great personal risks to bring us to this moment.

I believe it's important to acknowledge the elders and people who've long been in this struggle to recognize the human right to change your consciousness and heal yourself with powerful medicines, plant allies, and psychoactive compounds. In past years, this could have put you in prison, gotten your children taken away, or revoked your license to practice for those who were licensed professionals—people took great risks to speak out and oppose the drug war. And I think we should remember all the effort it took to get here. And also remember that people of color paid the highest price.

RM: *I wonder if there are things we haven't talked about that feel important to include?*

AO: Yes. Drug-checking is an essential service for psychedelic communities. It's absolutely essential for harm-reduction that people be able to access either the materials to check their own substances, or services that can do it for them. We know that there's a lot of adulteration and misrepresentation of psychedelic substances. That problem is escalated with the greater inclusion of compounds like fentanyl, which, if used improperly and sometimes unknowingly, can lead to overdose and possibly death. The stakes are very high.

I can't emphasize this enough: learn how to check your substances. Make sure that whatever it is you're ingesting is not misrepresented or adulterated in a way that can essentially poison you or someone else. Weigh your compounds out before you get to the event, batch them in specific quantities, and label them accurately. Don't inadvertently overdose on your friends. And always think twice before accepting substances that you have not tested yourself or were tested by another trusted person.

We made a decision in our own community to work with groups like DanceSafe to provide harm-reduction, education, outreach, and drug-checking services. They give out fentanyl test strips and teach people how to check their substances. They also provide other drug-checking services at our events. This is an absolutely essential service.

This is a message, especially for community leaders and event producers. Offer those services at your events. Go to the venues that you work with and make it clear that these are essential harm-reduction and community safety services. Work with your medics to make the importance of this message clear. Stand up for your community. Be courageous.

We should not judge people for the substances they choose to consume. Some people choose to consume fentanyl, Adderall, nitrous, and other substances that some people who prefer plant-based substances sometimes look down on. We should not demean people if their means of altering their consciousness is different than ours. I think that we should all support people's right to change their consciousness and support their ability to do that as safely as possible. We should not make judgments between "plant communities" and "those other people"—that's a false distinction, in my view. We are all in this together for personal and collective liberation, self-knowledge, and healing.

Remember that generations of chemists have been developing new molecules to provide psychedelic experiences. And that those experiences and those molecules are no less important and profound than plant experiences. Molecules are the building blocks of nature.

In our Take 3 community, we have many amazing people who make great art, music, and move the community forward in important ways. I think we understand that there needs to be balance within communities. That women, trans people, elders, and people of all backgrounds need to be empowered directly, to make sure that we are holding a safe container in a way that's empowering for the benefit of everybody. Being willing to engage in that discussion, that back and forth is what's required to build real communities.

Conclusion

I believe it is possible to weave the practice of deep community into our lives as a habit rather than only a response when surviving or in times of crisis. Intergenerational living, cooperatives, shared land projects, community organizing, home groups, and food justice are just a few expressions. Psychedelic communities can be containers for transformative experiences and places to integrate the insights received.

At its best, community can function as a driver of culture—an incubator for new ideas and expressions; solutions to what we are facing; spaces to process grief, rage, and joy; a place for our humanity to shine and be acknowledged; and a container for transformative experiences.

CHAPTER 6

Power

I feel like my whole life has been a study of power. I lived in a highly controlled environment, ruled by a long list of things my four siblings and I were not allowed to do: date, have our ears pierced, wear makeup, wear fitted or revealing clothes, talk to boys on the phone, and so on. And this was in addition to the thick holy book that pastors interpreted every weekend as even more rules for living. I felt unbearably constricted by the powers that be; even the name Rebecca means "to bind." Still, I was fairly laid back and even-tempered—until confronted with scenarios I believed were unjust. These were the only times I could really access my anger.

What infuriated me so much wasn't just witnessing or experiencing situations that were wrong or unfair; it was the way those with power (in my experience: parents, teachers, and pastors; and later as I became an activist, institutions and dominant groups) held and protected that power at all costs. It was the way rules and policies were unevenly applied to my peers and me, and the unapologetic response that seemed to say: "Deal with it. Might makes right."

As a young person, I dealt with this rage by rebelling. I soon learned that outright rebellion and outbursts weren't effective; they resulted in punishment and an even heavier hand of control. So I set out to outsmart the adults around me. I got good grades, in spite of skipping classes to smoke weed in the park. I broke petty rules and laws without getting caught. I looked for pockets of my life, however tiny, where I could experience agency and feel like a sovereign human being. I felt power when I was making my own choices about where I went and how I spent my time. I felt power when I started making my own money (even learning the hard way not to waste it all on teenage shenanigans). I felt power when I moved out at seventeen and my life didn't fall apart.

In the psychedelic field, the topic of power has been front and center, and I often have had feet in multiple worlds. I've experienced the ways those who are agreeable and embrace the status quo are rewarded, while those who speak out or break ranks are silenced or delegitimized. I've been asked outright not to say things in public forums that, while completely true, could disrupt the success of certain projects and efforts. I've engaged with funders and donors who have so many strings attached to their money that it's not worth taking. I've witnessed power brokering to a degree that I've never seen before—not even in megachurches.

It wasn't until I grew older that I realized power exists on a spectrum, and that I was much closer to systems of power than I had believed. You see, the power we each hold exists at a variety of intersections. It is not only dependent on one's unique circumstances (for me, being in a strict household and a religious environment); it also depends on one's proximity to the dominant social group. For example, as a light-skinned person, I have many powers and protections as I navigate the world that my Black and brown peers do not; my ethnicity is usually treated as something that makes me "interesting," rather than threatening.

As a young woman, I lack certain powers that are held by men and middle-aged people. As a cisgender, straight-passing queer person, I have the power to decide when and how the world will experience me as queer. As an able-bodied person, I have the power to comfortably navigate a world that is designed to accommodate me. As a working-class person without generational wealth, I do not have the economic powers of influence that my financially privileged peers do. As an English-speaking and articulate person, I am more likely to be heard in predominantly white environments and have my ideas taken seriously. These are just a few examples of how power shows up in every moment.

I've chosen to regularly interrogate my own relationship with power. I've realized it's not enough to hate those who have power; we all have it, and we have been conditioned to use it to participate in a culture of dominance. When we don't have models for the healthy use of power, we run the risk of misusing the power we gain. I've had to become aware of the ways I was wielding the power that came through my privileges, personality, achievements, and increasing visibility and influence over the course of several years. In my attempts to get free from oppressive structures, there will be ways I unconsciously repeat those same dynamics in my life.

A lot of my learned habits have had to change in recent years in order to earn the trust of the people I serve. The more power I'm entrusted with, the more important it becomes to not only have a personal practice of awareness, but to surround myself with people who will hold me accountable. I must also create structures in my spheres of influence that support checks and balances, power sharing, and group decision-making. Our world needs more servant leaders. I believe this is how we "fight the power." In actuality, we fight the abuse of power by healing our relationship to it. Power isn't going anywhere—it's part of being alive.

Defining Power

Power is a huge topic. There's just no way to adequately unpack a topic so big. And yet, power is an unavoidably present and profoundly impactful force in our societies, relationships, and medicine experiences. At its simplest, power is the ability to influence or control. We may hold power due to the roles or titles we hold, the responsibilities we've been assigned, or the privileges we've been born with.

Temporary imbalances of power are common in our world and can be part of healthy, dynamic communities. We are not each responsible for the same things at the same time. However, power structures designed to protect the power of certain groups or individuals at all costs and prevent access to power for others, are symptoms of a deeply unwell society.

Exploring Power

Many of our associations with power involve its imbalance, misuse, and abuse. We don't have many cultural reference points for the right use of power—that is, power that is generative toward collective well-being and thriving; power that is shared. More often, power is used as a tool to dominate and exercise one's will over others. Power is all too often hoarded, brokered, and exploited.

If power is the ability to influence or control, financial wealth is one of the most recognizable forms of power. It represents the ability to control not only one's own destiny, but also the destiny of the society around you. The extreme concentration of wealth and power we face, particularly in the United States today, creates a system of scarcity. By consolidating resources, people with access to and control over resources have wildly inordinate influence over those without access.

The ways we relate to power illuminate what we believe about the world and our place in it. For example, if we participate in hyper-competitive systems, this points to a belief that there are not enough resources for all of us to succeed and thrive. If this were true, it makes sense that humans would embrace individual power as the highest goal. Amassing individual power is an antisocial trait. It creates distance between oneself and the community. It pushes others down to lift oneself up.

In her brilliant book *The Power Manual,* author and nonprofit consultant Cyndi Suarez explains that the concept of difference is central to interactions and relationships of inequality. She states:

> The supremacist approach to power offers two options for dealing with difference: ignore it or view it as a cause for separation. A liberatory approach views differences as strengths and entertains interdependence as an option. For the dominant, embracing difference requires one to face one's fear of the subordinate, the other, and allow oneself to be changed, grow, and redefined by one's encounters.[1]

In the natural world, competitive dynamics are kept in check by a diverse ecosystem of interdependent and collaborative beings. While each creature is primarily focused on the continuation and survival of themselves and their kin, there is also a limit to the ability to hoard power and energy. A squirrel might store away for winter but creatures in nature rarely take more than they actually need or can use. A plant remains dependent on the sun and soil for nourishment, and never ceases to fulfill its "social contract," by returning oxygen into the atmosphere and nitrogen to the soil. There is no insulating oneself from the vulnerability of the shifting seasons, the ebb and flow of abundance. In the natural world, there is no ability to hoard so much that other species do not have what they need to survive. That is a uniquely human phenomenon. In a healthy ecosystem, all beings are held in balance through the web of life.

POWER AND LAND

In contrast, humans have broken our intimate links with our environment that sustains us (to varying degrees: Indigenous communities remain far more deeply connected than industrialized peoples). This fracture has been occurring over millennia. The question is, why? Perhaps as our awareness and control of the world around us increased, our tolerance for the vulnerability of participating in natural systems has diminished in equal measure. In time, we sought to outsmart nature by drawing boundaries on the earth and claiming ownership over it. Defending it with weapons. Growing our food instead of gathering it. (Although I admit that many creature comforts we enjoy today are a result of this shift.) We all participate in this separation because it is what we were born into and what we know.

Sadly, this separation from a vastly abundant and generous earth has created massive inequality between the haves and have nots. It has created barriers between us and the ability to meet our basic human needs—for food, shelter, safety, community, and belonging. To grossly oversimplify: those who have land have wealth. Those who have wealth beget more wealth. That wealth continues to rise upward and concentrate among fewer and fewer individuals who take little to no responsibility for the commons—the earth—while the rest of us face ever-increasing climate catastrophes against which those with wealth can insulate themselves.

We have created a situation where all life on earth is now impacted by the human pursuit of attainment of material wealth, power, and perceived security. It's a dire state of affairs. To share power and resources is to live in harmony with the laws of nature. However, this way of being requires trust in one another and in the earth to continue providing for us, in season and out. Somewhere along the way we abandoned our trust. I am not a historian, but this probably happened as the societies we created got bigger than the small tribal communities that allowed for real relationships. As a result, we have set out to create a sense of security by hoarding and capitalizing whenever we have access to resources, and opting for individual preservation rather than the health and well-being of the whole.

So, why are we talking about land?

The land and our bodies are the sites of our hope, pain, identity, and memory. These are the sites where power is abused and trauma occurs. Many of us live on lands that are not our ancestral homes and/or have ancestors who displaced its original stewards. In order to understand what we are healing, we need to understand where we have been, what has been wounded, and what we are healing toward.

The land we call home is relevant to every single one of us, not just those who identify as earthy or outdoorsy. Part of healing the wounds is healing our loss of connection to this marvelous planet that provides for us. If you eat food, you have a relationship with the land. If you bathe in water, you have a relationship with the land. If you take walks or have a pet or appreciate a sunset, you have a relationship to the land. If you have a child who hasn't been separated from their wonder and awe at the natural world, you have a blessed relationship with the land. These might not be strong or healthy relationships, but they are important relationships nonetheless; they are connections that impact one another.

Until we heal our relationship with the land, our healing will be incomplete. In the process of healing our relationship with the land, we begin to uncover the ways power is intertwined with all of it. We can remember what has occurred, become honest about the wounds the land holds, and in allowing ourselves to feel this we can make space for grief and take steps toward repair. The land holds memory. As we reconnect with it, we can chart a path to healing from the injustices that have taken place upon it.

What does all this have to do with power? Consider that the earth is one of the greatest powers we will ever interact with. We are small yet intelligent creatures, painfully aware of our own smallness. This used to inspire awe, love, and spiritual practice. But now, it seems we are living in denial and have spent generations doing whatever we can to assert dominance over the earth.

It makes sense that we have such complicated relationships with power. At an existential level, we aren't secure, and we can't seem to tolerate that. I believe the pursuit of power is related to the pursuit of security and gratification. It is the avoidance of the vulnerability and discomfort of the human condition.

Noticing these dynamics opens us up to explore and remember ways of holding and sharing power that are better for all of us. When we stop dominating and hoarding, we have a chance to experience true belonging. We no longer see others as a threat to our safety or the excess we are protecting. We can come to understand openness, transparency, and power sharing as the vehicle toward our security, rather than a threat to it.

POWER IN PSYCHEDELICS
Leadership Dynamics

As has been discussed, the psychedelic field is a microcosm of the culture in which it is situated. Long gone is the fantasy that we somehow exist outside of mainstream culture and its problems. In our case, this means the field reflects the cultural values of a competitive and domineering society. This means we have a unique set of challenges ahead of us: we are looking to engage with powerful substances to help heal wounds related to misuse of power, while holding our powers responsibly to not enact further harm. It's a spiral path that's difficult to simultaneously disentangle and walk.

Our use of power within psychedelics is linked with our experiences of power in society. For example, how might a person who has never experienced race-based violence respond if a friend or client expresses grief or pain from living under these conditions? How might a straight, cisgender-identifying person who has not spent time reflecting on their relationship to sexual orientation or gender identity respond to a friend who expresses uncertainty about their gender identity during or after a psychedelic experience? How might someone whose material needs were always met respond to someone expressing that their healing would be better helped by universal basic income than talk therapy? These are just a few examples of the many ways that minimization, dismissiveness, and unaddressed prejudice can retraumatize people seeking healing. Taken a step further, how will decisions about who and what we fund in the psychedelic space address or recreate systems of exclusion and oppression?

In Conversation with David Bronner

I spoke with David Bronner about the use of power within the psychedelic field.

David is the Cosmic Engagement Officer for Dr. Bronner's Magic Soaps. In addition to his support of advocacy for regenerative organic agriculture, David directs Dr. Bronner's resources to support animal advocacy, wage equality, and drug policy reform. One of his passions is the responsible integration of cannabis and psychedelic medicine into American and global culture. His activism embodies the company's mission—which encompasses a commitment to making socially and

environmentally responsible products of the highest quality, and to dedicating prof-
its to help make a better world.

David was born in Los Angeles, California, in 1973 and earned an undergrad-
uate degree in biology from Harvard University. He is a dedicated vegan and enjoys
surfing and dancing late into the night.

There are few companies that have done more for drug policy reform, fair trade labor standards, and environmental issues than Dr. Bronner's. Over the years, I have witnessed David navigate numerous tricky situations with humility and curiosity. I wanted to hear how he holds the responsibilities of having major power and influence, while staying authentic and committed to personal growth. I asked him how he thinks about the right use of power, especially when under pressure or when there aren't clear-cut answers.

"I believe true, responsible power is about empowerment," David said. He continued:

> It's about how you lift up the folks around you and power up allies who are doing awesome work. We need to be thinking about how to forge the coalitions needed to address the big challenges we're facing collectively. Leading is not always easy. Sometimes you get situations where you just need to step in and handle things, but more often, there are ways to reach solutions without being heavy handed.
>
> Part of being a healthy leader is exercising the power you have in a good way, especially in times of crisis or upheaval, to try and bring harmony to the overall situation. Sometimes you have to make really hard calls. The principles are simple: try to be fair, give second chances, and respond in proportion to the situation. I'm not some perfect Zen master about this, far from it. But I try to hold the samurai principle to never draw your sword in anger. It means we should aspire to wield our power consciously and only use it when needed. Don't overdo it. Use your power fairly. Consciously.

The importance of inner-work is multiplied for those who find themselves in positions of leadership, influence, or authority. Even with the best intentions to share power and practice justice, we must surround ourselves with people who can see our blind spots and bring them to our attention. The more power someone has, the more important it is that they have an inner circle of people willing to have difficult conversations and keep them accountable, and safeguards to protect those in proximity who are impacted by their choices. "My coach is someone I turn to a lot," David explained.

> The habits and intensity I've long relied on have, on the one hand, served me in many ways. But on the other hand, I discovered that they could impact my staff and my fellow leaders of the company in ways that were not always

positive. For example, what I viewed as "passionate intensity" could come off as domineering and angry, and interfere with the psychological safety necessary for our team to feel comfortable offering their best ideas, or letting me know that mine weren't so good. This is a hard reality to face.

So I have to stay committed to working on myself. I have gotten feedback in facilitated settings where my team has said, "Hey, dude, sometimes we're not sharing what we really think because of the way you're showing up. The environment doesn't feel safe." And I couldn't have seen that on my own, because it's not how I was perceiving it at all. So I need to be willing to make that effort to work on myself in that way. For me, that means getting less intense. And I think the team would tell you it's getting better. But I always have further to go.

Those of us who hold positions of leadership and responsibility need to take steps to mitigate the risks that come with that power. This can include training on right use of power, accountability and repair, as well as our own continuous inner-work so we can become familiar with our shadows and the parts that will get activated when we are depleted or stressed. It is also helpful to connect with leaders we respect for mentorship and support. But remember, even strong leaders are imperfect and bound to fall short; that is to say, don't put your role models on pedestals. And don't let anyone put you on one, either.

Power in the Medicine Space

Power differentials vary widely within the psychedelic field. Power is not just about the level of influence you hold; it also speaks to the responsibilities you have and the authority you have (or don't have) to intervene in situations. While one way of practicing is not necessarily superior to another, it's wise to be aware of the inherent differences at play when entering into a given context where psychedelics are involved.

The *guru/devotee dynamic* has a large power gap. This hierarchical system can lead to group cohesion, but concentration of power in one or a few leaders can create vulnerabilities that make abuse possible. Examples from beyond the psychedelic field illustrate how prone to problems these hierarchical systems can become for seekers who find themselves following a single leader for wisdom, guidance, and space-holding.

The *guide/psychedelic therapy* dynamic contains a significant power gap. Because many people are new to psychedelics and coming from a Western model that paints doctors, therapists, and psychiatrists as authorities and experts, many people are accustomed to handing their power to the professional and passively receiving treatment or guided therapy. The problem is that no one can be an expert on someone else's inner landscape and psychedelic experience. The client is truly the expert and the only one with firsthand experience. Everyone is unique and will respond to even the most predictable substances with variety. So I believe static or external expertise in psychedelic therapy is kind of a myth.

The *peer support dynamic* is not prescriptive and affirms the sovereignty and direct experience of the client as the authority. The facilitator serves in the role of a doula/helper to ensure safety and provide abiding presence and care. This is a less common power dynamic in our society, so it takes intentionality in navigating the nuance and clear agreements around responsibility and decision-making processes. The benefit is that clients are empowered with options throughout the experience, check-ins are frequent, and the client has the final say.

This helps prevent misunderstandings, oversights, misuse of power, and potential harm. Sharing power with the client disperses responsibility while upholding clear agreements. I believe that this dynamic has the potential to be the most healing since we are in a culture where many of our wounds relate to being overpowered, harmed, or controlled. A dynamic in which the client is empowered with choice, encouraged to trust their inner healer, and guide the process with safeguards not only creates an environment where psychedelics can have maximum benefit, but the meta experience itself can have healing properties.

FOR JOURNEYERS

Spend some time taking stock of your relationship with power. Can you locate memories of power being used responsibly or in a supportive way? How about times when it was misused to control, manipulate, dominate, or exploit? In what ways are your personal sources of pain connected to power? It's important to get in touch with these things so you can articulate what feels relevant to your facilitator.

When interacting with a prospective facilitator, take note of how your body feels and your behavior changes. Here are a few questions to help guide your exploration:

- Do you light up and speak openly or do you feel more reserved when speaking with them?
- Do your heart and nervous system feel settled and at ease or tense and alert in their presence?
- Do they express curiosity and ask questions that make you feel heard and valued?

Discomfort or lack of immediate chemistry may not be a sign that someone is unsafe for you to work with; however, there may be unconscious power dynamics playing out that will join you in the journey space. Take note of any "yellow lights" that arise. Choose a facilitator you feel a natural rapport with and who you believe has a healthy relationship with the power of their role.

FOR FACILITATORS

In many ways, power and responsibility are two sides of the same coin. They tend to increase in tandem with one another. Holding space for someone experiencing altered states is a major responsibility and comes with a great deal of power due to the journeyer's inherent vulnerability.

Power is not just about associated harms. Spend time getting clear on what the good use of power looks like in the session room.

- What formative experiences have you had with power and control? Can you think of healthy and difficult examples from your own life?
- How have your experiences shaped your beliefs about power?
- How do your beliefs about power shape your philosophy and approach to psychedelic healing?
- In what ways does holding power enable you to do your job well and keep your client safe?
- How might temporary and consensual power exchange actually be part of a reparative process?

Some power is essential for the role of a facilitator, but more is not always better. Get clear on the dynamics discussed above, and be explicit with your potential clients about how you work. As part of the intake process, spend some time discussing your approach to power and the intentional steps you take to manage the power differential.

Cocreating a plan for the session with your client is a practical and impactful way to build trust and set yourselves up for success. A client going through a journey they helped design can foster a sense of security. Honoring premade agreements during the session builds trust and enables deeper healing processes to take place (it is also an ethical mandate).

More about agreements and session planning will be discussed in chapter 9, on Consent.

In Conversation with Bob Otis Stanley

I met Bob while collaborating on an Oregon psychedelic decriminalization effort called the Plant Medicine Healing Alliance. We quickly discovered that we held a kinship and natural alignment in personalities and our orientations to leadership and life. Through this, a mentoring friendship was formed.

I was honored when I founded Alma Institute and he agreed not only to join the board of directors, but (thanks to my pleading) to hold a seat as interim board chair. I needed someone with a wealth of board experience to help coach me in the early seasons of Alma's development. I wanted to speak with someone who holds societal power and privilege, who I see humbly working to share that resource for the collective good. He agreed, but emphasized that he was eager to be replaced by someone who comes from our priority communities.

It became a running joke among the board that we should rename Bob's position to "Reluctant Board Chair," because he would repeat during roll call at each meeting that he was eager to vacate the position as soon as we were ready. It prompted plenty of laughter, but this willingness to share power also strengthened the team. A bit about Bob:

A mystical experience at age seventeen led Bob into a lifetime study of sacred plants and substances. He has explored soul-healing entheogenic work for over thirty-five years, independently and with his father, family, and friends, learning from traditional and Western teachers. Explorations in Guatemala, Brazil, Mexico, India, Jamaica, and elsewhere were dedicated to healing practice and learning. Personal and group experience leads him to a careful and respectful relationship with what he believes to be Sacraments.

Bob is senior pastor at Sacred Garden Community Church, was the founding chairperson of Decriminalize Nature in Oakland, and is a cofounder of the Sacred Plant Alliance (SPA). Bob's plant work and life science research have generated many public talks and over fifty publications. Following psychology and religious studies degrees from UC Santa Cruz, Bob earned a master's in divinity from the University of Chicago; and engaged in postgraduate work in sociology and cognitive science at New York University.

RM: *What do we mean when we talk about power in the psychedelic field?*

BOS: Broadly, I think we humans are still trying to figure this out! Understandably there is a lot of concern around access and exercise of power in this field. There are different ideas about what power means, and about how power relates not only to realizing shared goals, but also how it relates to conscious or unconscious corruption, domination, exclusion, and harm.

These different ways of thinking about and working with power are really important. There's power as control or domination, meaning power as the capacity to make whatever I want to happen, happen—independent from and even at times against others' interests. This reflection of power is authoritarian—associated with, for example, domination by institutions such as corrupted religion, colonialism, racism, and sexism. But there's also a different kind of power, which would be power as the capacity to achieve shared goals. This power stems from knowledge, even from wisdom. It requires listening to others and being able to communicate in a power-neutral manner; to be aware of positionality, contextuality, and their critical impacts in order to learn, grow, change, influence, and align interests.

I want to propose that by its proper definition, authority is good, desirable, and useful. Authority is legitimate when it starts with listening, when it is sensitive to and seeking to elevate and learn from the authority of others, when it recognizes the impact of its own power, position, and privilege even when listening. Authority is legitimate when it aligns with shared goals and when it brings the experience, insight, and capacity to support meeting those goals. A good teacher brings wisdom and authority, to help me realize my own goals within this lifetime.

RM: *In that light, the associations that come to mind for me are expertise and eldership. I believe these things are connected with authority. That it can be something earned, that represents wisdom and the holding of something sacred or important. The idea that responsibility comes with authority.*

BOS: Yes. Unfortunately, this respect for our wise elders is something we've lost in the United States largely. I believe in part it's because we have experienced so much authoritarianism from the Church, from government, from alienating economies, from patriarchal structures, whatever it may be. So in contrast to authority, authoritarianism is not coming from a place of insight or wisdom. Authoritarianism, associated with the effort to control without regard to independent agency and spirit, hurts us. It causes distrust, and disintegrates us and our communities. It may be important to note that a sense of responsibility can also lead to fundamentalism and domination when we move from arrogance and fail to listen to others.

Neo-fundamentalism in the psychedelic space is a big risk right now . . . there can be more than one form of good practice! Let's develop our good practice but be open to forms of practice that may be different. Let's avoid bringing domination into this field—whether from fear, control, narrow concepts of rightness, or fundamentalism.

RM: *How do you see authoritarianism and fundamentalism connected?*

BOS: A great way of growing authoritarian power is to say: "I (took a course, or learned from this Taita, or . . .) know something and you don't know it. And if you don't do things the way I say, you're gonna go to hell or be harmed or punished or are illegitimate in some way."

So authoritarianism and fundamentalism are often really closely associated.

But there's a whole different set of paths that lead into authority. And that is experience. Experience of shared or persistent effort over time to achieve shared goals, learning what works and what doesn't work in community. This is the grounds for developing authority: being together in community, engaging effort with reflection, to realize shared goals. This grows authority through experience. This also defines eldership, which we've largely lost track of in the United States as well.

We suffer under leaders who don't understand the value of authority itself. So then we're like, "Fuck authority, we don't want any power in our lives." We don't want any knowledge or wisdom or experience. And then we just get total trash, we just get junk! This is a recipe for unconsciously growing authoritarianism. So—it's important that we get clear on the distinction between power as domination (authoritarianism) and power as wisdom to align with and support facilitation of shared agency and goals (authority). There is a difference between power as domination and power as insight and capacity to realize positive outcomes in community.

RM: *So I'm hearing that we've conflated useful forms of power with domination. How do we start to repair or rebuild trust in the holding of power?*

BOS: It's possible to identify things to avoid in forming and exercising power, almost by process of elimination. Am I listening with discernment to my own and others' power and position (e.g., critically)? Do I know the community and issues being engaged personally, from direct experience over time? Are my own interests transparent to those I am engaging? Am I moving from a place of relative humility and willingness to self-reflect?

RM: *Setting up structures for accountability is so important: we can't rely solely on our good intentions or highest ideals, we need to make sure we are not immune to critique and accountability processes. So that if I go rogue, those around me have the pathways and resources to intercept that.*

BOS: Openness to learning is one key to legitimate authority, which is to be capable and willing to self-reflect and learn. At the same time, communities need to support leadership when it recognizes its own fallibility. Demanding perfection doesn't allow for the learning that authority requires! It's an exciting space, and a challenging one. An ideal setting for growing power can be mutual mentorship within caring, respectful, trusting community; growing integrity; and wisdom together.

There's much more power in learning and exercising aligned values, even with the extra effort needed to reflect diverse views. This holds much more power than unilaterally saying, everybody has to think like I do and act the way I insist. Do it my way or I will destroy you!

Another important thing that is happening in the psychedelic space to be aware of is neo-fundamentalism. In my opinion, if anyone is asserting that they know *the way that it all has to be,* that's probably already corrupt. It could be a training program or a community of practice or what have you. But this work is evolving.

If we claim esoteric knowledge as if it is indisputable, that's a pretty transparent, unconscious way of claiming power. If someone says, "I just know some things you can't know. This is the only right or good way to practice," we should take note of that. This is one of the biggest risks in the psychedelic space right now. If we say everything has to be the MAPS or the CIIS [California Institute of Integral Studies] way, the Decrim Nature or the Shipibo or Mazatec way, that's not really authoritative; I think that's authoritarian.

I'll end by saying that we need to be super careful about how we use our power in efforts of Indigenous reciprocity. It really does need to come from relationships and listening. We can't just exercise our colonial power to heal all of the problems of Indigeneity and colonialism. You see how that's contradictory? Sometimes, we just have to slow way, way down. We need to quietly look and listen and let the next action become clear to us. We don't need to be hypervigilant heroes trying to intervene on everything. Sometimes we need to focus on our own healing or on healing within our community, and allow folks to do what they're gonna do rather than trying to exercise all of our power over everyone, everywhere all the time.

Conclusion

In order for our healing work to be truly worthwhile, we have to get clear on how we participate in, benefit from, and uphold power structures that can actually inhibit the healing of other people. We have to become aware of and invested in tearing down and transforming these structures. If we do this work, a whole world of possibility opens up to us. It is my hope that we will use the inquiry within this chapter to help us reflect on and heal our own relationships to power. I believe this is at the heart of healing and whole medicine.

CHAPTER 7

Pacing

Not long ago, I was invited by a mentor to sit in ceremony with a medicine circle a few states away. I'd had the time carved out in my schedule for a program I was no longer participating in, and I had been feeling due for some good medicine, as it had been almost a year since my last deep dive. I agreed to join.

Because flights were so expensive, I decided to turn the week into a solo road trip, something I do often. I thought the open road and shifting landscapes would be good medicine in themselves, offering me a chance to prepare for the ceremony and let go of the spiritual and emotional detritus of modern life before arriving.

The amount of driving required that for several days I wake early and drive all day to make it to my next campsite by dark. My optimistic self disregarded what a ten-hour driving day feels like. I took moments by the rivers and ponds, pulling over to give something to the land every time I crossed into a new territory. I watched the birds of prey circle for their next meal, savored the stillness of small towns, and collected roadside flowers to press in my journal.

I arrived to a warm, familiar face. My mentor and I had one day before the ceremony, in which we slowed down to soak in some healing waters and spend some much-needed quality time together.

The ceremony itself was profound. It was a good kind of struggle at first, mostly somatically (which I'm sure was partially due to the amount of sitting I had put my body through on the previous days). Once I passed through the difficulty, I experienced a night of communion that has been truly unmatched in my life. It felt like, for once, the labor and striving of my being fully ceased. Awed presence and belonging were all I knew, as though I was sitting at the feet of a beloved grandmother while she braided my hair and spoke reassuring words in my ear. I let myself fall in love with life again and I was given the reassurance and strength to carry on the hard work in a good way.

The other details of what was given are between myself and Spirit. As the sun rose, we fell into a cradled sleep. A few hours later, after the ceremony had been closed, we packed up our things and parted ways. I had to get on the road; I had miscalculated my days and realized that in order to be back in Portland to get my son on time, I needed to be in Utah by nightfall.

The first few hours of driving were okay. I was technically sober enough to drive; however, anyone can attest that the days after a big ceremony should be spacious and restful. Instead, I was in a hot metal machine speeding down the freeway. Still so energetically open, I had to take extra measures to insulate myself from the "default" world. I played meaningful music, worked with guardian plants, continued to honor the dieta (a special diet and lifestyle protocol intended to support preparation and integration of medicine work), and found secluded rather than crowded places to rest when I could.

By afternoon, I was seriously regretting my choices. It was a shock to the system to cover hundreds of miles of billboards, drive past dozens of dead animals, and witness landscapes shaped by aggressive industry. Instead of the beauty I had witnessed on the trip down, I was confronted with the ways we are ravaging a precious home in order to enable our imbalanced, extractive lifestyles. "This is why we can't have nice things," I thought.

By sunset, I was trapped in Salt Lake City rush-hour traffic and extremely fatigued. The fading skies and headlights were impacting my vision and I started to feel like I was living through a real-world nightmare. Several exits were blocked due to road work, so I had to weave through construction sites with blaring floodlights and crowded work crews in search of my place to land. Meanwhile, the medicine circle was settling into their second night of ceremony, which I had decided to miss due to scheduling constraints.

When I finally arrived at my rental (a moment I thought might never come), I felt disoriented and afraid. All my systems were asking what had just happened. I did a small clearing ritual, took a long shower, and FaceTimed my partner. I slept fitfully, woke exhausted, and put air in my tires for another long day on the road.

This trip was a lesson learned the hard way. The medicine I received on that trip was a powerful blessing. However, I believe it was a disservice to the medicine, and some of the benefits of the experience were lost because I didn't create an environment in which they could settle. If you don't have the space for proper preparation and integration, it's advisable to take steps to rearrange your schedule so you do. If that's not possible, consider postponing your participation so that you can be fully present before, during, and importantly, after the experience.

Defining Pacing

I define pacing as the practice of regulating the intensity and frequency of psychedelic experiences.

The practice of pacing requires that we take note of our inner states and honor natural rhythms of expansion and contraction innate to life. Working with psychedelics is an expanded state, and while profound and beautiful, too much time spent in this state can inhibit our ability to participate in everyday life. When taken to an extreme, this lack of tethering can result in problematic use, or even psychotic breaks.

Pacing affords us the time to absorb the benefits of our experiences and implement the changes they inspire. It comes with numerous benefits. I believe it is essential to the future of this field and is something I feel is not adequately discussed.

Exploring Pacing

We live in a culture that says more is better. Is that true with psychedelics? We have plenty of cultural reference points that suggest *no*. I see psychedelic experiences the way I see salt: while some is good, more isn't necessarily better, and there is *certainly* such a thing as *too much*.

Not only can pacing enable us to get the most out of our experiences, it can also be a harm-reduction measure. While relatively small, there is a risk of (re)traumatization that can occur if people uncover too much material too fast. This is especially true when working with high dosages or new substances. It can happen whether folks are consuming casually for personal exploration or the express purpose of deep healing. On top of the potential for accessing difficult biographical material, existential insights can be intense and sometimes range from destabilizing to disturbing. This is why support for ongoing integration is so central to psychedelic work. We can't prevent every negative outcome.

Pacing is one simple measure we can take to prevent a shock to the system. We do this by being intentional with our own habits, how we engage with the people we serve, and the messages we convey to the general public.

PACING IN THE WORLD

So much of the harm being done in the world is bound up in the culture of urgency. Urgency is a symptom of Western, white supremacist culture, which values productivity above all, and fears the scarcity of time and resources. When we move too quickly, we do not leave room for reflection. We do not believe we have time for process or to reconsider. Moving quickly means that existing power structures are preserved because we never stand still long enough for us to see them for what they are.

Uncoupling this urgency from our healing environments is crucial. We are human beings with animal bodies and tender nervous systems. Our psyches are not machines to be repaired as rapidly as possible; we are creatures who need spacious processes that allow for the unwinding and unraveling of pain and trauma.

A world that honors pacing is a world returning to our inherent wisdom. Because we live in a globalized, capitalist society, we will not always be able to slow down to the degree that is just. But we can create microcosms of spaciousness within our realms of influence. Again, what happens at the micro level will eventually ripple out and shape the broader culture in which we are situated. We can help one another by giving the permission, reminders, and accountability to slow way down. Catch our breaths. Bask in the beauty and unknown of the in-between moments.

In the words of Somatic Abolitionism founder, Resmaa Menakem: "Slow down. You. Have. Time."

THE BENEFITS OF SLOWING DOWN

GROUNDING IN LIVED REALITY. This relates to the very real issues of spiritual and psychedelic bypassing. When engaging with psychedelics, we often face the temptation to flee more and more to the world of altered states. It is understandable, especially when we find respite from the dire status of the modern world. Escapism can be good medicine in certain moments, but ultimately risks disengaging from our full lives and relationships and developing a preference for altered states. Guides talk about "high-chasers" and "blisstronauts."

ROOM TO BREATHE. Developing a sincere, ongoing practice has as much to do with the space between sessions as the profound insights received during sessions. It is our role as journeyers and facilitators to support whole-life healing, not just psychedelic experiences. This can mean ensuring there are meaningful support networks before and after, reflecting on whether now is an ideal time for a psychedelic experience or whether there might be other lifestyle changes that would prove beneficial first, and encouraging the person to take ample time between journeys to rest and digest.

CONSERVATION OF MEDICINES. Psychedelics are not infinite resources. Every substance, whether a mushroom, a cactus, or an MDMA rock, took resources to produce. There is reverence to be found in being intentional with one's consumption. When we approach psychedelics with gratitude and recognition of their precious nature, this energy comes into the session with us. If we come from a consumer mindset that we can have as much as we can afford, we may not be as intentional about our use and could eventually tilt into overuse.

MEANINGFUL INTEGRATION. Within traditional Indigenous practice, individuals' entire lives are integrated with medicine. When the whole world around you is seen as sacred, ceremony is happening constantly, in seemingly mundane moments as well as intentional containers. So there is no reducing an experience into the compartments of preparation, session, and integration. With an intact relationship with the mystical, the practices of integration such as chanting, drumming, storytelling, dance, spirit manifestations, and ritual cleansing occur before, during, and after the ingestion of entheogenic substances and also do not rely on the psychedelic experience. They carry weight on their own.

In this way, although intentional containers are created to mark the opening and closing of major ceremonies, traditional medicine work is also a discipline without clear beginnings and endings. The profound experience is nested within a social fabric that holds a shared history and cosmology and carries established practices and supports for meaning-making.

A strong argument can be made for the importance of integration. Consider the amount of unstructured use that is reported as not particularly healing or meaningful. Many of us have spoken with people who report that they "took mushrooms in college, and it didn't cure my depression." Put another way, the substance itself doesn't carry the power to transform. It is a blend of the substance, intention, context, preexisting factors of one's life, follow-up care, and action that all contribute to the potential impact of a psychedelic healing experience.

One benefit of the medical model of psychedelics (as opposed to the recreational one) in modern society, as presented in the research and clinical trials, is its emphasis on structured integration. In this context, integration is woven into the treatment protocols and seen as an essential phase of the healing process. In these contexts, integration usually consists of "integration therapy," which refers to working with a trained therapist skilled in working with patients who have had psychedelic experiences. These sessions help the client unpack the material uncovered during the experience and draw meaningful connections. It might also involve helping the individual chart next steps for moving forward with these new insights. *This doesn't have to mean drastic, sudden life changes; in fact, that would be antithetical to integration. The therapist or facilitator can support the person not only in making meaning from their experience, but also in slowing down when the impulse arises to make major decisions on the heels of a big journey.*

In nonmedical contexts, there is a lot more flexibility in the ways we weave insights from our journeys into our default realities. Intention and integration hem in the psychedelic experience on the front and back ends. Before a session, spend time getting clear on the reasons for partaking. Ideally, this intention setting can coincide with a protected period of time that is free of (or reduced) tech distractions, socializing, and consumption of mind-altering substances.

While it can vary widely and should not be limited to what is explored here, some practices are commonly relied upon to assist with the integration process. These are not unique to the psychedelic experience; they are practices that are often already mainstays in a person's life and continue after the psychedelic experience. These can include:

- Expressive, somatic, and mindfulness practices such as art, writing, dance, movement, meditation, and time spent in nature.

- Working with professionals such as talk therapists, bodyworkers, acupuncturists, nutritionists, or traditional healers from your lineage.

- Rest and quiet time spent with loved ones who know you best. Integration doesn't have to feel like work; it can also be nourishing and joyous as we start to find new ways of being that are reflective of our true, more healed selves.

Pacing in the Medicine Space
FOR JOURNEYERS

Take stock of your consumption habits and ask those close to you (inner circle or the facilitators you work with) to provide feedback or observations about your patterns of use. Consider the following questions:

- What does integration look like in your life?

- Can you recall examples from your life when you did not effectively integrate an experience? What was the outcome?

- When invited to sit in a circle, are you more likely to accept or decline?

- What are your reasons?

- How can you tell when the insights of the medicines are weaving themselves into your life?

- How do you know when you are ready for another ceremony?

- How do you gauge what dosage is right for you? Do you tend to be conservative or to go big? Why might this be, and what would it be like to have a different dose than you prefer?

- Are there integration practices you'd like to explore that you haven't tried?

- Who can you rely on to give you honest feedback about your consumption of psychedelics?

FOR FACILITATORS

As a person who journeys, you should spend time with the above questions. It is important that we model for our clients the habits that can support them as well. In addition, spend some time reflecting on the way you conceptualize pacing and talk about it with your clients. You might consider using the previous prompts for journeyers as starting points for conversation with prospective clients.

- What standards do I have in my practice for making decisions around dosage and frequency?

- Do I have an incentive for my clients participating in more frequent ceremonies?

- If so, how do I hold this tension? Who holds me accountable to not "oversell"?

- How do I navigate situations where I don't believe my client is ready for another (or a first) psychedelic experience?

- What responsibility do I hold in supporting my clients' integration processes?

- What additional resources can I provide for my clients to support their ongoing healing process beyond what I can provide?

In Conversation with Aaron Orsini

I originally met Aaron while working together on an equity committee within the psychedelic ecosystem. His leadership role actively serving neurodivergent communities is nothing short of trailblazing. I've always appreciated his practical outlook on mind-altering substances, and the way he approaches public education from a balanced, fact-based framework. He moves with humility, integrity, and a refreshing dose of humor. In addition to his many contributions to this field, Aaron is also a guest instructor at Alma Institute.

Aaron Orsini is an autistic author, educator, and researcher of psychedelic medicines. He is a research coauthor partner to University College London, where he's collaborated with researchers on academic studies exploring psychedelic use among autistic individuals. He has also published three books related to this area of focus—Autism on Acid, Autistic Psychedelic, *and* Introduction to Psychedelic Autism. *Additionally, he helped establish AutisticPsychedelic.com, an online hub for connection, education, research, and support for autistic adults, their family members, and the professionals who seek to serve them through various forms of psychedelic practice.*

RM: *Pacing is something you and I have discussed several times. It's something we don't really talk about a lot in this field.*

AO: I agree. And I think that's largely due to the cultural emphasis on the "one and done" approach. Typically, clinical research has been structured that way, mainly because of limitations related to validating cost-effective approaches. Also, there's something to be said about people being new to psychedelics and being so blown away by a single session that they claim tremendous progress right away, only to realize that they've only just begun the real work of ongoing integration. There's always more work to be done. As someone who aspires to live a psychedelic-integrated lifestyle, I feel compelled to speak to the less-often-discussed ways of weaving psychedelics into the rhythms of our lives, in subtle and regularly scheduled ways, as a sort of "mental hygiene" routine.

First, we need to look at the established framework that views these substances as intervention tools or tools of healing. I think if we lived in a culture with more expanded and routine access, and more normalization of that same access, then we might start to view psychedelics as something more like diet supplements, or preventative medicines—tools that can help us stay in harmony with our hearts, and listen to our hearts more continuously, the same way that a deep meditation practice might.

RM: *What do you see as the relationship between pacing and integration?*

AO: They're super connected. Having a preexisting support network, like an integration or support circle, can really help to fill in the gaps between major session work. Self-inquiry is great, but we're also social creatures. Showing up to be of service is a great way to work on one's personal mental health as well. The way that we do this in our Autistic Psychedelic Community is that every Sunday, we come together. It's not always necessarily about integrating a psychedelic experience, but it's definitely about having group accountability and having the chance to check in with peers about our progress, victories, setbacks, etc. Because, again, no matter how many psychedelic sessions we have, we generally have to return to this plane of everyday awareness. And when we do, it helps to surround ourselves with those who have traveled to some of the same mental or emotional highs and lows.

I maintain this complex dance of compassion and accountability by surrounding myself with people who support me *and* challenge me. In this way, I'm always processing a lot of this stuff. And I think the psychedelic community at large is composed of those who can understand the importance of this type of deep discussion. In our Autistic Psychedelic Community meetings, we foster these conversations by providing that type of space, and reminding the community that that space is always there if they need it. We also have other connecting points available, like our text-based chat groups and forums, where community members can seek out support at any time, from anywhere on earth, at the tap of a few keystrokes.

It's integration, but it's daily life. And we're normalizing the idea that we can be radically accepting of messy emotions. And because we're healing with others, it feels a lot more accessible and sustainable, as opposed to only ever being able to be authentic in the brief amount of time we spend inside of a therapist's office.

RM: *I'd love to hear how you see the relationship between dosing and pacing.*

AO: I think largely because of the insistence upon the medical model having more of a leaning toward standardization—and that includes standardization of things like dosing protocols—that the intuitive approaches get left out of the picture. And I think that yes, precision medicine has outstanding potential, but so does our ability to cultivate intuition with demonstrably safe medicines like psilocybin.

People often ask me, "How do you do your microdosing?" And honestly, there are some baseline beginning points, but then everything else arises from intuitive variation, and depends so much on the particular context. It's like if someone were to ask me, "What's my coffee protocol?" then I might say, "Well, it's not that rigid. What am I doing? Am I trying to stay awake? Does my day require a quiet mind or a quick mind? Do I need this or that substance to help me focus? Would twenty minutes of exercise be just as effective? How about meditation?" After asking myself questions like this, in a gut-check sort of way, I then make a determination of dosing (or not dosing), factoring in not only the number of washout days that've elapsed since the last dose but *also* the task I intend to engage with on that day.

The same goes for dosing with moderate or larger doses of something like psilocybin. Yes, there are some standard protocols, but rigidity toward dosing approaches also has its edges. We don't need to give every first-timer three to five grams of mushrooms as though that's the only way to begin. And we don't need to give everyone microdoses every three days either. Instead, I'm proposing the continued push toward systems that allow for dosing variability, all while still remaining within the bounds of what we know about these compounds in terms of general safety and tolerability.

It's a shame, really, that medicines like psilocybin can't be cultivated legally or brought home legally just yet. Because legal cultivation models and other similar approaches allow for the exact state of nonurgency that people really need in order to settle in and feel okay with making realistic, incremental changes—at a pace that also feels stable, and safe, over time.

Conclusion

Integration is lifelong, and I believe it builds in layers. If we think of our lives as a rich compost pile, psychedelic experiences can dump a lot of new, nourishing material onto us to process. Over time, these gifts become more and more blended into our lives and identities so they are indistinguishable from who we are. Those experiences never disappear; they become part of us. If we add too much too fast, we're prone to making short-term messes in our lives or we'll, at the very least, need longer to process and restore balance.

I have found that the longer I work with the medicines, the smaller the space becomes between my default reality and the realms of the medicine. Sometimes, working with tobacco, cannabis, or meditation carries me into psychedelic spaces where I can pick up where I left off. The gift of years of practice is that the medicines become like familiar friends, such that I can sense them more clearly and tap into the entheogenic space with more ease. For me, this means that when I am moving slowly and living intentionally, I can settle into a subtle and continuous dialogue with them. When this happens, I feel called to consume them less frequently and in gentler doses when I do.

I believe the real opportunity lies in a paradigm shift where we stop separating psychedelic experience from integration and stop separating integration from life. If we can relate to the journey as not having a defined beginning and end point, then we can view the days and months leading up to and following our journeys as gradual unfoldings of that experience. Integration no longer becomes something that we "do," separate from the rest of life, but a natural process that plays out with the support of our attention and a series of habits and micro-actions. Slow, steady, and intentional use supports lasting shifts in our lives, and can be an expression of reverence for the substances that make this all possible.

CHAPTER 8

Harm-Reduction

I was once asked to speak on a panel at a grassroots psychedelic conference. I also coordinated a few scholarship spaces for community members I was connected with. One of them was a young woman new to the scene, who had experienced profoundly healing benefits from working with psilocybin mushrooms and wanted to connect with the community. She rode the bus from the next town over, thrilled to attend.

At the event, there were numerous booths set up, and among them was a vendor selling mushroom microdose capsules. In spite of the legal prohibition against selling mushrooms (even in places where they have been decriminalized), many enterprising groups have created craft products and began offering them to the community in recent years.

I was returning from a lunch break when I was called to the green room. The event organizers explained that the young woman had taken a "microdose" she had purchased from one of the vendors and she also smoked some cannabis with a group outside during an intermission. They had told her the mushrooms were "super light," that she "would barely feel it." When I arrived, I found the guest sitting with a trusted colleague during what appeared to be a nervous breakdown. She was wide-eyed and withdrawn, and began asking me repeatedly if something bad was going to happen. The others intuitively left the room as I tried to reassure her and sort out a plan. I sat with her for a while as she rode waves of various emotions—crying, overwhelm, and fear. She began to apologize repeatedly, in between moments of asking if I was going to hurt her. I reassured her she had nothing to be sorry for, that I was a safe person.

It was clear that the paranoia was increasing, so I mentally ran through my options: try and call someone she knew to come get her, wait with her on-site and see if her anxiety subsided, or offer to drive her home. After some deliberation, I offered to take her home. She agreed. She was hesitant to get in my car, so I resolved to be as patient as needed and I channeled my safest "mom" energy. I explained the exact plan to her: that I would put her address in my GPS, drive her home, walk her to her door, and leave once she was safely inside—as long as she didn't need my company and was comfortable with that.

On the half-hour drive, she oscillated between asking if I was going to kidnap her, to laughing about how silly the situation was, to apologizing and expressing embarrassment. I let her know again that I was more than happy to support her and

I thanked her for trusting me. I reassured her that no one at the event was judging her. I shared a story about a time I passed out from cannabis overconsumption at an industry event and had to have my partner come get me. We had a good laugh and this seemed to ease her worries. Once she was settled safely at home with her partner, we stayed in touch via text over the next twenty-four hours and I did what was within my capacity to support her in processing the experience.

I felt an element of responsibility, having invited her to attend the event, unaware of what risks might be present. I also felt that the event organizers could have done much more to set community agreements around consumption of substances on-site, and ensure vendors were aligned on harm-reduction and risk management best practices. This was a woman who had a major trauma history and, preventably, had difficult memories that surfaced in a nonideal setting. While decriminalization has many benefits, we never know the histories people are holding. It is risky to promote consumption of powerful psychedelics to strangers in unsupported settings, and especially problematic when a financial benefit can be gained from their consumption.

I hope we can find ways to embrace decriminalization through a harm-reduction paradigm that holds that we are communally responsible for educating, managing risks, and taking care of each other when challenges arise. Psychedelic event organizers should be aware and prepared for these events to occur, and as attendees we should hold organizers accountable to have harm-reduction plans in place and keep the community informed of these offerings.[1]

Defining Harm-Reduction

Harm-reduction is the practice of compassionately minimizing risks associated with certain behaviors, rather than trying to prohibit people from engaging in them. The best practices of harm-reduction emerged out of activism within drug use and sex work communities.

In psychedelics—even with our best intentions around discernment, and awareness of power dynamics, pacing, and creating optimal settings in which to consume—the real world is full of imperfections. As the embrace of psychedelic substances continues to increase, so too should our skill set around supporting risk reduction in less controlled environments.

FRAMING HARM-REDUCTION

We do risky things every day. It helps to take an honest look at our cultural attitudes toward harm-reduction; and our individual underlying beliefs about the types of behaviors that deserve harm-reduction and the types that we have an impulse to shun, reject, and punish. For instance, driving a car is the most deadly thing most of us do on a daily basis. Society has responded by creating laws about using seat belts, creating standards for car safety features, and public education campaigns to prevent distracted or impaired driving.

Many people choose to drink alcohol, which comes with an array of safety and health risks. Instead of criminalizing the use of alcohol (which was attempted from 1920–1933 with Prohibition, which carried a slew of unintended consequences), we have established social norms. These can help promote balanced alcohol consumption, require bartenders to stop serving when someone is visibly intoxicated, and discourage risky behaviors such as drinking and driving.

It is worth reflecting on why our society has deemed some behaviors worthy of harm-reduction measures, while forcing those who participate in other behaviors to the margins and the shadows. Does selectively outlawing activities that carry risk create greater community safety on balance, and how do you measure those benefits against creating a sense of moral superiority for those who only participate in activities legitimized by current law? Many harm-reduction and drug policy reform advocates argue that legality does not define morality. And that by transcending the legal structure for our only guidance on what is right, we can exercise our individual and collective discernment to embrace measures that are humane, compassionate, practical, and logical—legal status notwithstanding.

Harm-reduction is rooted in radical presence and acknowledgment of the behaviors that people actually engage in. Harm-reduction, at its best, is rooted in compassion and empathy. It means letting go of ideals or judgment, and pursuing good in the absence of perfection. It encourages small, accessible shifts in behaviors and habits and provides support for those shifts so the person can experience greater safety, agency, and dignity. To be a harm-reductionist is to provide support without trying to control, or "sitting, not guiding," as is commonly referenced in psychedelic harm-reduction circles. In that way, there is power sharing woven into the practice of harm-reduction, because it is built on the foundational assumption of a person's sovereignty and agency. They have the power over their decisions, and you are coming alongside as a support to possibly ease the burden and lighten the load, on their terms and with consent.

Exploring Harm-Reduction

Public discourse is becoming more favorable toward psychedelics. Yet, with more media attention we have less space for nuanced intricate conversations. Moreover, this specific discourse around altered states of consciousness has led to a fracture in our thinking, where certain substances are embraced as beneficial and others are rejected as problematic.

Psychedelics are not for everyone. There are real risks; adverse reactions do occur; and in order to have an enduring field of psychedelic healing, we need to be honest with the public and take a sober, balanced stance on safety and risk. When we are honest, we can take meaningful steps to mitigate risks and ensure the people choosing to consume consciousness-altering substances can have the best outcome possible.

Before we can talk about harm-reduction in the psychedelic and plant medicine contexts, it's important to understand and acknowledge the roots of the harm-reduction movement. Harm-reduction is not only about minimizing risks and maximizing benefits. It's more than that. In many contexts, harm-reduction is truly life-saving work that goes unrecognized and under-resourced.

For those who have come to this book from plant medicine contexts, this chapter may present a growth edge. We are going to talk about gritty contexts that aren't necessarily centered on healing and thriving and beautiful stories. We are going to talk about real-world challenges and how communities have organized themselves to survive and find ways to thrive.

Harm-reduction work has taken many forms and iterations since the 1960s. The roots of harm-reduction come from communities of people who use drugs and do sex work, and those who feel called to support and resource them. What these communities have in common is that they exist in the shadows due to criminalization. When people have to hide because of risks of arrest and incarceration for their activities, they cannot rely on public health services the way the general public can. As a result, communities of everyday people who face legal risks for their activities have organized themselves to help build community safety and well-being. There is beauty in the bonds of solidarity forged within oppressed communities—even under the heavy hand of injustice. These are the roots of harm-reduction.

Groups that have laid the groundwork for harm-reduction include the National Harm Reduction Coalition, the Drug Policy Alliance, the Young Women's Empowerment Project, and the Sex Workers Outreach Project, among many other grassroots and community groups who came before and have worked alongside them. Other social justice groups throughout the decades have operated parallel to and in solidarity with harm-reduction efforts, united by an understanding that those directly impacted by harmful systems hold the wisdom needed for resistance and change.

In psychedelic harm-reduction, we are fortunate to have groups today such as DanceSafe, the Zendo Project, Kosmicare, and many others dedicated to reducing the risks associated with experimental and recreational drug use. These groups stand on the shoulders of pioneers such as the Hog Farmers' "Please Force" at Woodstock (1969), the Grateful Dead parking lot medics, the Rainbow

Gathering CALM volunteers, Oregon's community care nonprofit White Bird, Rock Med concert medics, and the Green Dot Rangers at Burning Man.[2] Much of what has been learned in recent decades about psychedelic facilitation and the nondirective approach has roots in harm-reduction settings such as these.

Harm-reduction exists at the individual and community level, and includes not just physical harm-reduction and safety measures, but also emotional and spiritual harm-reduction.

PRINCIPLES OF HARM-REDUCTION

While there is no single, centralized definition of harm-reduction, there are a few key principles that most efforts are built around:

1. Individual sovereignty—all people have the right to choose what they do with their own bodies and consciousness.

2. Right to health and safety—all people deserve to have their health and safety protected regardless of the choices they make.

3. Intersectionality—the harms associated with risky activities are directly tied to marginalization related to race, class, gender, orientation, trauma history, and lived experience.

In her brilliant anthology, *Towards Bodily Autonomy,* author and healing justice practitioner Justice Rivera writes that "These wars on bodily autonomy are rooted in the gendered, racial, and economic biases that encode our country's DNA, supported by a constitution that has never evolved in a meaningful way."[3]

Later in the book, in collaboration with Shaan Lashun, they write:

> For as long as we can remember, queer and trans communities, communities of color, and our sex working and drug using ancestors have been mitigating the harmful consequences of slavery, colonialism, and imperialism. Harm-reduction practices are ancient and remembered, but the harm-reduction movement began as a public health and social justice movement in the late 1970s in response to a critical need to reduce HIV transmission.[4] The community response was condoms and syringes. The government's response was sodomy laws and the war on drugs—fearful measures that sought to eradicate communities in which supremacists' hate was already manifesting.

Examples of Harm-Reduction Services

The following is an inexhaustive list of forms of harm-reduction that have saved countless lives over the decades. Many of these remain in a fluid state of existence and must continue in their fight to operate due to continued stigmatization and misinformation.

FOR DRUG USERS

+ Drug-checking services
+ Drug-checking supplies
+ Safer drug use supplies such as needle exchange and free pipes (enables people to smoke heroin through a bubble pipe instead of injecting, which reduces the risk of infection and allows people to pace their intake)
+ Publicly and freely available supplies of overdose prevention measures such as Narcan
+ Safe consumption sites

FOR SEX WORKERS

+ Safer sex supplies
+ Community networks to let other sex workers know when someone has been harmed by a customer via date sheets
+ Worker unions

FOR PSYCHEDELICS

+ Real-time support line such as the Fireside Project
+ Support sites for difficult experiences at festivals such as the Zendo Project and Kosmicare

FOR ALL

+ Access to healthcare services that reduce stigma for drug users and sex workers
+ Free public education around options and best practices
+ Advocacy for more humane policies and decriminalization of stigmatized activities

Fractal Harm-Reduction

Beyond the foundational practices of harm-reduction within drug using and sex work communities, we can apply the principles of harm-reduction to micro and macro contexts. The benefits are consistent: more safety, consent, dignity, and humanity. We have models to look to within the psychedelic field as guiding lights, particularly the Full Circle Tea House that was the inspiration for the Zendo, and private groups that embody these principles at their gatherings, events, and in their communities in daily life.

It's important that as we expand the meaning of harm-reduction, we do not dilute or co-opt the original meaning and intent. In other words, we must never erase the marginalized communities and activists from which this valuable work emerged. We can work together to keep our language specific and be clear in what we are referring to as we seek to apply these principles more broadly throughout our society.

More wisdom from Justice Rivera and Shaan Lashun:

> Over the last 50 years, the concept of harm-reduction has grown from a set of practical, nonpunitive survival practices to a philosophy and framework applied to a range of public health and safety issues, including domestic violence and the COVID-19 pandemic. At its core is the understanding that shame is not a productive agent of change, and robbing people of resources only decreases their chances of survival. "Just say no" isn't as effective as "What do you need to be okay?"[5]

I strongly encourage you to get a copy of *Towards Bodily Autonomy* to support your learning. It is rich with history, insights, and invitation.

INDIVIDUAL HARM-REDUCTION. This is where most traditional HR (harm-reduction) practices land. This involves understanding and acknowledging a person's choices and providing support measures so they can experience the least harm and the most benefit. For this to be successful, participation needs to be voluntary and tailored to the individual's unique circumstances.

COMMUNITY HARM-REDUCTION. When someone is enacting harm within a group such as a social circle, spiritual community, or medicine circle, we can engage in community harm-reduction practices. This entails intervening in the situation in a manner that creates the least harm and the most protection/benefit possible. This is where harm-reduction and transformative justice are connected. Transformative justice is a potent form of harm-reduction because it begins with a clear-eyed look at an entire system that is creating harm. From there, it sets out to not only disrupt the active harm when it occurs, but also change the conditions so it's less likely to keep repeating itself.

SOCIETAL HARM-REDUCTION. When we all live under oppressive systems like extractive capitalism and all the other *-isms* that come with it, societal harm-reduction means minimizing the harmful impacts of these systems while acknowledging that we currently live under them. Practices all can participate in may include benefit sharing circles, mutual aid networks, exchanges, swaps, free activities, activism efforts, libraries, parks, barter fairs, warming centers, shelters, public art, education campaigns, and direct action.

Societal harm-reduction for psychedelic enthusiasts requires stepping outside of insular love-and-light paradigms and looking at the hard realities of the world around us. It asks that we engage with one's local community, understand the real-world challenges being faced, and embrace integration practices that extend benefit beyond individual growth toward positive impacts in your family, neighborhood, and locale.

I also consider policy reform and justice work an expression of societal harm-reduction. It is seeking to reduce and alleviate the damages caused by existing systems, while simultaneously working to dismantle and replace them.

ECOLOGICAL HARM-REDUCTION. This practice takes into account the web of planetary impacts caused by patterns of individual action, collective action, and large-scale policy decisions. It seeks to prevent and disrupt the most damaging actions (such as major deforestation, war actions, and systemic oppression) while divesting from these large-scale systems where possible and supporting on-the-ground interventions through relief efforts.

We can participate in ecological harm-reduction by supporting water and land protectors, participating in direct action, uplifting Indigenous-led initiatives, advocating for corporate accountability, and doing our part to build and support thriving regional food systems and less harmful energy and transportation systems. As with all forms of harm-reduction, it is important to understand that perfection is rarely possible and that the real world is full of contradictions and nuance we have to live with. When we weave these practices into our lives, we can find value in the smallest and most weighted practices. Soon, it becomes difficult to separate harm-reduction from ceremony. This is an expression of an integrated life.

For those in psychedelics, ecological harm-reduction can mean understanding how your medicines are produced and sourced and choosing options that are aligned with values of human rights, sustainability, and Indigenous sovereignty. More on this in future chapters.

Harm-Reduction in the Medicine Space

FOR ALL OF US

Always get your substances tested. There are various reagent test kits available online. Urge event organizers to host groups that can provide this essential service at gatherings and festivals. Create healthy peer pressure among your social circles to normalize drug testing, and model this behavior.

Tell the truth. Everyone's risks are unique, so create conditions where each person participating has as much information as possible about the experience and has enough time to make a grounded decision whether or not to participate.

Understand dynamics in psychedelic communities that have higher risk of harm. These can include hierarchical power structures that enable one or a few people to make unilateral decisions that affect the collective, experimental protocols that reduce the likelihood and ability of informed consent, and personality traits such as narcissism and savior complexes.

In Conversation with Dr. Angela Carter

I have been fortunate enough to collaborate with Dr. Angela Carter on numerous drug policy-related projects in Oregon. We worked together on the Oregon Psilocybin Advisory Board's Equity Subcommittee and I also consider them to be a dear friend and mentor. In addition to countless key roles within Portland's mental health, trans healthcare, and drug policy efforts, Angela has been an integral advisor and member of the curriculum development team at Alma Institute.

Dr. Angela Carter is a licensed Naturopathic physician practicing in the Portland area and a member of Oregon's governor-appointed Oregon Psilocybin Advisory Board. They are the founder and clinical director of the Equi Institute, a nonprofit healthcare organization focused on promoting the health and well-being of the LGBTQIA2S+ community of the Pacific Northwest. They also chair the Meaningful Care Conference, a biannual integrative LGBTQIA2S+ medical conference in Portland, Oregon.

Dr. Carter works as an LGBTQIA2S+ health advocate with several organizations including Basic Rights Oregon and Oregon Health & Science University to improve the culture of care for LGBTQIA2S+ people in Oregon hospitals and medical facilities. Dr. Carter teaches in a variety of settings: they have taught minor surgery, LGBTQIA2S+ health, and gynecology in medical schools; and have been a presenter on transgender health issues at national medical conferences.

RM: *Why do you think harm-reduction is so tied up with morality in our society?*

AC: Even if we aren't actively involved in fundamentalist religion, our culture has been shaped by puritanical values. So that results in an avoidance of anything that is pleasurable. Anything that is embodied and physical. It's a binary system, where you're either in the good graces of God or you are not, and it's a zero-sum situation.

We don't have to ascribe to that. We can acknowledge that we are each a facet of the universe, one of the faces of this amazing experience of consciousness, and we all have, at the baseline, a deserving to live and to thrive, even if we are not doing it "right" by someone else's standards. There's so much tied up in the idea that certain lifestyle choices make us discardable. That's just not true. We all deserve to live and have the opportunity to thrive.

I can look at someone and say: "Oh, it hurts when you do that. Let me help it not hurt so much." It means releasing control over other people. How freeing. Giving up the idea that you know what's best for someone else. We all know what's best for us at any given moment, even if it is not necessarily ideal for our bodies, our spirits, or maybe even our communities. We have the right to make whatever choices we need to make, to survive.

RM: *In many ways, the principles of harm-reduction are connected to the nondirective approach. They both center the intelligence and agency of the person you're supporting, and seek to reduce the perceived or actual power differential between people.*

AC: As I work with people, it's basically impossible for me to detangle the roles between the sitter and the person I'm sitting with. Even if I don't take medicine, just by sitting with someone and bearing witness, I am profoundly changed by that experience. I can't isolate myself as the facilitator separate from the client. It's not a one-way process.

So this whole idea of hierarchy, where I am sitting with you, I am the one who is in control of the situation and guiding you, I don't see it that way. In reality, I've also been guided by the people I sit with, in ways that are so profound. It's an exchange.

And I believe harm-reduction also holds a recognition of that reciprocity and interconnectedness. So I think it's important that we hold that reminder in this work, that it calls for humility. It is a privilege to walk with someone on their journey. And to know we are going to be changed along the way.

RM: *How do you see harm-reduction and collective healing connected? How can psychedelics assist these endeavors?*

AC: Here's something I learned as a physician that I think translates to this work for all of us. People's illnesses and symptoms cannot be separated from the contexts they grow up and live in. Access to health-promoting resources and services is not currently guaranteed to all people. Far from it. Harm-reduction is recognizing the system we all exist in, and how it creates harm to each of us individually and together, and actively trying to change that system. So we all can heal and be free together. It's the collective liberation piece.

And the same is true of psychedelic services. If someone comes in and is depressed, we need to take the time to understand the factors contributing to them being depressed. Of course, it makes sense that people are depressed, living in an environment that is not conducive to our humanity. It is so out of balance with the natural world, with our own nature. The systems of competition, scarcity, and domination are oppressing people, creating disease. It is holding all of us down.

And so, with psychedelic services, somebody might come to you who wants to address their depression. You can respond and say, "Well, this will change your brain biochemistry. Here's some psilocybin that will help a bit," and then they go home, back to the system you existed in previously. And, you know, maybe they'll feel less depressed for a couple of months. But it's going to come back because you're immersed in the same system.

We are a community, and we heal together. We cannot heal together if we don't address all of these pieces that are affecting the entire community.

RM: *For many groups, the Western notion of rugged individualism never fully took root because folks have had to rely on one another in order to survive. I think about groups like immigrant communities, Black communities, queer and trans communities, and groups that are neurodiverse or have disabilities.*

AC: I'm lucky enough to know this firsthand. I have been lucky enough to be a part of the queer and trans community, which is a deep community; it is a lineage. We have shared community together over the generations. It is not a genetic community, but we are a family. And we care for each other and love each other. We become each other's siblings, especially when our families have rejected us.

A connection and understanding of family outside of that patrilineal focus, the queer community is one representation of this, but there are more. Folks who are bonded by shared struggle. Think of Mad Pride, folks who are marginalized due to a DSM diagnosis. Groups of people with physical disabilities. Groups who don't speak the dominant language. Groups of racialized people living under white supremacy. Groups of working-class laborers.

I think the piece that is the most important in all of this is remembering and living into the truth that we are not isolated. We are all connected. We are linked to each other. And, again, our liberation is tied up in everyone's liberation. We need to act accordingly. These medicines can be a part of our individual healing and liberation, but what's most exciting is that this can ripple into creating a healthier, safer world for all of us and all living beings.

Conclusion

Harm-reduction is tied up with power and consent. Inherent in our quests for healing and liberation is the fight for sovereignty over our own bodies and minds. The practices of harm-reduction are real-world moves that hold revolutionary potential when applied more broadly. Bringing compassionate support to people without coercion, manipulation, or judgment is not only reparative in its own right; it also disrupts the puritanical notions that only some people deserve safety, health, or belonging. Respecting the dignity and humanity of all people is central to the work of consent.

CHAPTER 9

Consent

This topic is close to my heart. Unfortunately, most of my earliest awareness of consent came to me through its violation. I experienced multiple sexual assaults before I even reached adulthood, and my story is devastatingly ordinary. I didn't have a truly consensual sexual relationship until after I graduated high school. So I'm no stranger to the ways consent, power, accountability, and trauma are bound up with one another.

While the conversation around consent is often limited to the realm of sexuality, I've realized this is also part of the issue; it is relegated to a topic we are already reluctant to talk about. In truth, consent touches our whole lives and colors our day-to-day interactions in more ways than we realize.

I've learned a lot of reparative lessons around consent through being a parent. I am a very high-touch person who grew up in a low-touch home, so I have spent most of my adult life making up the difference. Babies can be awesome because they're such snuggle monsters. When my son was a toddler, he naturally began to gain independence and create more space from me. Still, I would mindlessly stroke the top of his hair when we were out and about, as a subconscious way to stay connected to him.

One day, while we were standing in the grocery store checkout line, he grabbed my hand and stopped me. He looked up at me and insisted, "Mom! I no am a dog. I no am a cat. Don't pet me!" The cashier looked at me and we both burst out laughing. He had put me in my place. I apologized and worked to break the habit.

During the pandemic, he was much older and we were cooped up during two years of distance learning. We invented a wrestling game called "Mom-a-gator." Essentially, I would trap him underneath me and he would squeal and fight and try to escape, but just as he started to get free I would catch him again. He thought we were just playing, and it was a chance for us to burn off steam. But it was also a chance for him to learn key relationship skills he'll need his whole life. (Parents are sneaky like that.) We set ground rules around touch. We made a safe word. We checked in frequently. Questions like, "Are you still having fun?" "Did that hurt?" and "Can you move your elbow?" became second nature. When we took things too far, we respected each other's "no" and apologized where needed. We built trust. We had fun.

It was healing for me to witness a young person developing the relational skills that I wish my peers and I had as teens. I believe a generation of people who embrace a culture of consent could change our whole society.

Defining Consent

Consent is a word that occupies various meanings and contexts. For the sake of this chapter, we're looking at consent within the context of psychedelic experiences, as well as a broader look at the interconnected web of systems where these experiences occur. This chapter is about personal and bodily autonomy, and touches on themes that may surprise or activate some readers. As always, the invitation is to take the time you need, notice how your system responds to the content, take breaks, and return when you are able. Consent is about choice. At its core, it represents the ability to choose what happens to you, and voluntarily agree to it.

I asked Emma Knighton, MA, LMHC (she/they), a leading educator on consent and trauma-informed care in the psychedelic field, to help define consent. In her words, consent is "the embodied process of cocreating an agreement centered on negotiations of desires, limits, and risk." They explain that, secondary to that definition, consent speaks to how we grapple with being in relationships while holding the reality that we are all capable of harming each other. We'll dive into a deeper discussion with Emma later in this chapter.

Before we proceed, it's important to acknowledge that much of the rapidly mainstreaming practices around consent were created and have been stewarded by the kink and sex work communities for many years. These are decentralized global communities stigmatized due to mainstream attitudes and judgments about relationships and sexuality.

Consent is absolutely critical when engaging in activities that hold inherent risk. In fact, the status of consent is a major aspect of what distinguishes pleasurable, choice-based activities from ones that can be abusive and harmful. Because of its importance, those who engage in kink and erotic labor have developed frameworks for navigating consent that benefit all of us who now draw from them. These groups coined the terms SSC (Safe, Sane and Consensual), RACK (Risk-Aware Consensual Kink), and the Four C's (Caring, Communication, Caution, and Consent).

As we aspire to establish our own useful frameworks for navigating consent within psychedelic contexts, it's important to give credit for where existing tools originated and the people who have carried the torch for bodily autonomy in a period in history when it is under threat.

Exploring Consent

GUIDING PRINCIPLES

While entire books have been written about consent, here are a few guiding principles we can lean on for our purposes:

1. Consent is specific.

2. Consent is given freely and voluntarily.

3. Consent is active. It can be withdrawn or changed at any time.

4. It is impossible to give true consent under the influence of a mind-altering substance.

CONSENT AND OUR BODIES

Our bodies are the landscape where life is experienced. They are the places we discover, practice, and integrate the meaning of consent, violation, healing, sovereignty, and agency. They are the sites where great harm is stored over generations, and where the most sublime experiences of being alive often take place. What we come to understand about consent and our bodies can and should be applied to our communities, other living beings, and the land we belong to. It can extend inward, too, to apply to our internal emotional, spiritual, and energy bodies, where practices of consent are equally important.

Humans are high-touch creatures. We are mammals, kin with bears, chimpanzees, horses, and dolphins. Before we connect through words, ideas, or shared activities, we connect through physical contact. There is a transfer of energy, intention, and emotion when we touch one another. Touch can convey safety or danger. It can be used to harm or heal. Touch is so important and foundational to our well-being that the absence of it during infancy can result in failure to thrive, weight loss, stunted growth, and in extreme cases, even death.

We are being taught from our earliest days in life about touch, sensation, pleasure, connection, and safety. Depending on our context, we can learn that touch is safe and comforting, or that it is dangerous and harmful. Most people experience many kinds of touch and pick up mixed messages about consent as we grow up. Small children are often physically handled, moved, and redirected in order to keep them safe. As they grow, children are then often urged to hug or kiss relatives, even when they don't want to. As adolescents we experience classrooms, dress codes, religious environments and sports, along with sex, drug, and food education that dictate what we can and should do with our bodies. Some youths endure bullying, policing, and abuse. All of these experiences shape the ways we inhabit our bodies and the strategies we develop to be safe.

As a culture, we often equate sensuality with sexuality, which is a missed opportunity. We are sensual beings by nature. We relate to our environment using our physical senses of touch, taste, smell, sight, and hearing, as well as the more enigmatic forces of energetics and intuition. One of the hallmark traits of plant medicines and psychedelics is their profound and amplifying effects on the senses. They cause us to temporarily experience the world differently, and these shifts are often reported to have lasting effects on one's sense of connectedness, belonging, and well-being. Because psychedelics can amplify sensitivity, it is all the more important to be extremely intentional with how we approach touch and all the other sensory and extrasensory elements involved with a psychedelic experience.

While most of this chapter is about navigating touch and personal sovereignty within a psychedelic context, it is impossible to have these discussions with integrity without looking at the ways consent and consent violations exist in our history and our human experience more broadly.

Consent and power are inextricably linked. Most, if not all, atrocities in human history hold at their core a consent violation. As discussed throughout this book, these traumas echo in our bodies and nervous systems and affect the way we live and move through the world. Communities are forced to develop survival strategies that prioritize safety from violence, at the expense of thriving, rest, community power, and cultural expression. While these structures hurt all of us, we are each affected differently based on our social locations and our proximity to the dominant group. The Wheel of Privilege and Power,[1] popularized by Sylvia Duckworth, is a useful tool to help us look more closely at our intersecting identities and the ways they impact our lived experience under these power structures. I invite you to take some time to become familiar with it and consider where the various aspects of your identity fall on the wheel.

As a result of historical and continued violence, much of our healing work must take place in our bodies. This is the site of the trauma and the healing. This is why so many great leaders in social justice, especially Black feminist leaders, discuss the body in their writings about liberation—from Audre Lorde, bell hooks, Sonya Renee Taylor, Sabrina Strings, Toni Morrison, Octavia Butler, and James Baldwin to today's adrienne maree brown, Prentis Hemphill, Tricia Hersey, and Resmaa Menakem. Accessing safety, resilience, and pleasure in our bodies is a practice that takes a lifetime, and it is an essential part of our collective efforts to heal, get free, and live differently. Those of us working in healing spaces today hold a great debt of gratitude to the aforementioned leaders, and so many among, before, and after them, who, by necessity, have held intimate knowledge of the inner workings of liberation and healing over generations.

In her book *The Politics of Trauma,* author Staci K. Haines, cofounder of the generative somatics training program, writes that we must look to social justice as the *primary prevention* of trauma, while also acknowledging how essential healing from trauma and oppression is to that goal, to decreasing suffering and to increasing safety, belonging and dignity. If we do not understand and integrate the shaping power of institutions, social norms, economic systems, oppression and privilege alongside the profound influences of family and community, we will not fully understand trauma or how to heal from it. We will not understand how to prevent it.[2]

As we approach healing with psychedelics, it's imperative that we take the time to develop a foundational understanding of how trauma exists in our bodies, trauma's relationship to consent, and how they are inextricably linked to the healing process. Psychedelic experiences can exacerbate traumas or set healing processes in motion. This awareness can help us develop practices that support the latter.

CONSENT AND PSYCHEDELICS

As discussed in previous chapters, the dynamics that have played out on a global scale have shaped us as individuals and communities. As a result, we see in the psychedelic field the same themes of power imbalances, lack of consent, and urgency we see in almost every other movement or field of practice. In order to stop repeating the same harms, we need to unlearn damaging beliefs about power and consent and settle into more healed ones.

Consent as a culture ripples throughout life and asks us to transform how we approach pretty much everything. It touches our relationship with nature, with ourselves, and with how to meet our needs without harming others. We can learn from healthy ecosystems that live in this constant state of nonverbal negotiation, which results in balance and homeostasis.

CONSENT FROM ORIGINAL STEWARDS

One of the uncomfortable truths that we hold in this field is that we are here because of historical consent violations. Rarely, if ever, have entheogenic medicines been introduced to non-Indigenous communities in the context of permission and consent. We will discuss this at length in chapter 12, on Reciprocity.

CONSENT FROM THE MEDICINES

What does it mean to ask permission to partake?

Many traditions teach that the medicines have their own consciousness, whether plant medicines, sacred brews, mushrooms, or even lab-derived substances. This is why we talk about establishing a relationship with them. A consent-based relationship involves invitation, sharing, listening, care, and a balance of give and take.

Fortunately, we don't have to reinvent the wheel; we can train, apprentice under, and collaborate with groups across disciplines beyond the psychedelic field. This way, we can take cues from those who have spent time on critical analysis and developed protocols for working with sacred plants and the communities. who steward them. Consider leaders such as Vandana Shiva and Winona LaDuke, and frameworks like the Nagoya Protocol. This is an internationally upheld set of standards for consent-based use of genetic resources that protects biodiversity, promotes benefit-sharing models, and prevents exploitation of Indigenous peoples for their traditional knowledge and expertise. The United States is one of the only countries in the world that has not signed the Nagoya Protocol.

The principles of the Honorable Harvest, as popularized by Robin Wall Kimmerer in her book, *Braiding Sweetgrass,* can guide our way of sourcing and utilizing medicines. She writes:

> The Honorable Harvest, a practice both ancient and urgent, applies to every exchange between people and the Earth. Its protocol is not written down, but if it were, it would look something like this:
>
> Ask permission of the ones whose lives you seek. Abide by the answer.
>
> Never take the first. Never take the last.
>
> Harvest in a way that minimizes harm.
>
> Take only what you need and leave some for others.
>
> Use everything that you take.
>
> Take only that which is given to you.
>
> Share it, as the Earth has shared with you.
>
> Be grateful.
>
> Reciprocate the gift.
>
> Sustain the ones who sustain you, and the Earth will last forever.

Though we live in a world made of gifts, we find ourselves harnessed to institutions and an economy that relentlessly ask, "What more can we take from the Earth?" In order for balance to occur, we cannot keep taking without replenishing. Don't we need to ask, "What can we give?"[3]

CONSENT AS RELATIONSHIP

I spoke with Courtney Watson, LMFT, about how consent is a central part of whole medicine.

Courtney is a licensed marriage and family therapist and trained psychedelic-assisted therapist who has founded a ketamine clinic at Doorway Therapeutic Services, focused on providing psychedelic therapy to queer and BIPOC clients by queer and BIPOC providers. She has also started a nonprofit, Access to Doorways, to raise money to ease the financial burden for queer and BIPOC clients looking for psychedelic therapy by queer and BIPOC providers. She shared the following with me.

Connected to consent is the investigation of relationships. We all need to be looking at our relationships to other cultures. What is my relationship as a Black person who is descended from enslaved Africans, and also descended from Chahtah in the Mississippi Valley? What is my relationship to whiteness as someone who is also descended from white folks who brutalized both of those communities? What is my relationship to Korean folks, when we have this history of racial strife because of riots in the 1990s as someone who is a mother to children who are also Korean?

What is my relationship to culture and my positionality around that? What is my relationship to the plants? What is my relationship to the flora and fauna that surround me? I have this big cedar tree next door that is dropping sap on my car all the time. So what is my relationship to that plant? If I bring cedar into a ceremony, what relationship have I cultivated with the spirit of that plant in order to do that?

As facilitators who are thinking about consent, we need to think about our relationships. All of these aspects of what we bring into the ceremony, including the culture of the person, their ancestors, the plants that we use with them.

I met someone who was serving medicine and talking about opening a space with white sage. So I brought up that I think we need to acknowledge that white sage is over-harvested and is part of Native tradition here on Turtle Island. I asked, are there plants from your lineage as a white person that you can bring in, such as rosemary? It is also a really good plant to bring in: it's not over-harvested and it's easily available. And this person said, "No, I have a right relationship with sage. I have five hundred bundles of sage drying in my room."

If you're going to bring white sage into a ceremony to clear the space, or you're gonna bring tobacco into a ceremony to protect it, what is your relationship with that plant? What about the people and bioculture it comes from? Did you receive consent to harvest it or did you purchase it on Amazon? Did you pray over this plant and are you conscious about your relationship with that plant before you use it?

To me, consent extends beyond the session. It means deeply investigating my relationship with every aspect that happens in that ceremony before I do it. So that I can share what's needed with the client, so that they can also consent to the ceremony that we are cocreating.

CONSENT IN PRACTICE

Navigating consent is not a static, boring thing. Consent is a living, breathing place we arrive at together. It is relationship. It is a vehicle for our liberation. Consent is the result of active participation and navigation, time for reflection, and space for emergent shifts in real time. Much of the unease around consent culture is that as a society, we have either never developed, or have long forgotten, what it means to be in a reciprocal relationship built on deep listening.

Due to cultural context, Westerners often approach our interactions from a transactional perspective rather than forming agreements based on the agency and sovereignty of all individuals and the good of the whole. Under transactional pressures, consent is no longer an empowering exploration shared by multiple individuals; it becomes reduced to a way of preventing liability.

However, when we take the time to reframe the idea of consent from a liability lens to a possibility lens, everything shifts. Now, instead of consent being a box we must check in order to prevent lawsuits or misunderstandings, it becomes an exploration that offers wide-open horizons where first and foremost, the client can experience being empowered, heard, trusted, and respected. In addition, the facilitator can rest in the knowledge that they have supported their client in a way that centered active choice.

Safety Planning

As we've discussed in previous chapters, there are several discussions that need to happen and core agreements that need to be made before embarking on a psychedelic experience. Among these are:

1. What is the journeyer's relationship to consent? Is there anything the facilitator should know about past experiences that may shape the agreements that are made?

2. What substance is being consumed, in what dosage, and who will be sourcing and providing the substance?

3. Are there any medications being taken that could interact with the substance? If so, has the client's healthcare provider been consulted and what steps will be taken to reduce risks?

4. How will you navigate touch? What kinds of touch are okay, and in what context?

5. How will offers for touch be communicated and agreed upon during the experience?

6. Spirituality: Are the facilitator and journeyer on the same page about the spiritual elements of the practice, and what agreements are there regarding how spiritual phenomena will be handled?

7. How will a physical health emergency be handled?

8. How will a psychological emergency be handled?

9. How will harm be addressed if it occurs?

10. What mechanisms are there for reporting or providing feedback?

These are all items that need to be addressed ahead of time, with plenty of space for the client to ask questions; and for all involved to set clear boundaries and expectations and arrive at a place of agreement. This process of navigating consent is a critical step, especially for newcomers and those working with a space holder for the first time. It not only provides important groundwork for the medicine session; it also provides enough time and space for everyone involved to notice if there are core misalignments in the approach or expectations, and address them.

Agreements made during preparation take precedence over agreements made during a psychedelic experience. These prior agreements create the outermost boundaries we can move within. In order to establish and maintain trust and surrender to the experience, the client needs to know that their requests will be honored regardless of what might emerge during a session or how connected with their default reality they are. These boundaries can certainly close in during a psychedelic session, but we must avoid expanding or renegotiating them once a substance has been consumed, as *it is impossible to give full consent while under the influence of a consciousness-altering substance.*

Navigating Touch

A wide spectrum of touch can occur during a psychedelic session. Touch as a technique within a healing modality requires training and navigation, as we discuss in this chapter. Touch used in safety or logistical procedures (such as helping someone get to the bathroom or assisting them in repositioning themselves within the room) should still be used consciously and with consent whenever possible.

In Betty Martin's book, *The Art of Receiving and Giving,* she unravels the complexities of what she calls the "Wheel of Consent." In short, the four quadrants of the wheel provide a framework for understanding both the action that is being taken, and whom it is for. It is divided into Serving (touching someone for their benefit), Taking (touching someone for your benefit), Accepting (being touched for your benefit), and Allowing (being touched for their benefit). Within psychedelic sessions, *all touch should take place for the client's benefit.* Most often, this will fall into the Serving category—this could mean holding a client's hand, ankles, or shoulder for grounding, placing an arm around them, or providing a shoulder to cry on.

Unlike within Betty Martin's training contexts, in the real world, touching and being touched cannot be so clearly separated; technically speaking, to hold someone's hand or to give them a hug is also to be touched yourself. So the filter becomes: Is this touch for the benefit of the client? Is it initiated, requested, and/or welcomed by the client? Has it been agreed to ahead of time? Touch that can be erotically activating for either party should be strictly avoided in these contexts. While this varies from person to person, generally this includes positions that involve full body contact or contact with erogenous zones such as the mouth, neck, chest, abdomen, armpits, lower back, thighs, buttocks, and genitals. The more detailed the agreements made beforehand between facilitator and client, the more trust can be built and the less risk there is of consent violations to occur or be excused after the fact.

Premade agreements are just the beginning of navigating consent. The real work happens in real time, as it is important to develop the skills of checking in with oneself and one another. The facilitator must have the capacity to say, *"How is this for you?"* and adjust their approach based on the client's feedback. Does the client feel comfortable enough to say, *"That doesn't feel helpful"*? What other nonverbal cues could be designated ahead of time so the client can stay immersed in their experience and still communicate with the facilitator?

Touch for Safety

Cases of escalation and crisis management are beyond the scope of this book; the facilitator should have a plan ahead of time for how to respond to rare cases of agitation or aggression. The use of physical restraint should only be used by trained and qualified professionals in cases where the physical safety of the client, facilitator, or others cannot be achieved any other way. If a facilitator is not trained and qualified, they should remove themselves from the situation and get help immediately. At this point, everyone's physical safety becomes the top priority, and unfortunately, consent becomes much more complex and difficult to navigate.

This is why creating as many explicit agreements as possible ahead of time is important. It is ideal that the client can consent to emergency safety plans as well as other forms of touch. Harm-reduction groups such as Boom Festival's Kosmicare, MAPS' Zendo Project, and X Razma's Guide for Guides have more thorough guidelines around how to safely navigate cases of escalation.

Spiritual Consent

There are widely varying perspectives on what is actually occurring during a psychedelic experience. This is something we can't know for sure; mystery and wonder are notoriously elusive to human systems for measurement and documentation. For some, the sensations and impressions are simply a result of disorganized brain activity, and the visitors and visions one encounters are merely constructs of the human brain.

However, many others believe that accessing hidden realms with the aid of plant medicines and psychedelics can transport us not only deep into our own psyches, but also into other realms and planes inhabited by living entities beyond oneself. These could be understood as God, Source, the Universe, the collective unconscious, spiritual entities, ancestors, and energies of all kinds.

Because of the various cosmologies you'll encounter in the psychedelic field, it is important to spend enough time with a facilitator to find compatibility before embarking on a journey. Alignment in belief systems can help ensure that the right conversations take place up front and that there are no surprises for either party when it is too late to turn back.

I asked Courtney Watson to talk about the importance of spiritual consent.

Most of the time informed consent is lacking around spiritual consent. I remember once I was in a holotropic breathwork workshop. I was not provided accurate information about what I was entering into. There was someone that was clearly struggling with a spiritual entity of some sort. We were in a group setting, and I was not aware that that was even a possibility. It felt really violating. I felt like I did not consent to being in a group where someone could be struggling with some demons.

Fortunately for me, my ancestors had guided me to put together a bag. I brought some Agua Florida with me among other things. I was able to protect my space and the person I was partnered with, who was the breather during that session. But I didn't consent to that. So I think informed consent means providing as much information as possible of what could happen. People in this field aren't talking about Spirit. They might vaguely reference, "You might see something scary; go toward it." But what does that mean? Training programs aren't talking about a lot of the really "strange" things that can happen. And the result is that clients and sitters are experiencing things in real time without full preparation. And that is a consent violation.

Many ceremonial traditions have specific protocols about how to open and close a space, which is often referred to as the "container." This is a spiritual and energetic practice of sealing up a space with protection from outside energies so that the journeyer—who is opening themselves up to a vulnerable state, often for the purposes of healing or insight—can fully embrace the experience without interference from unwelcome outside forces. A facilitator should be prepared to share with their clients about their worldview and spiritual orientation, so agreements can be made about how the session will be conducted and the client has a chance to consent.

In connection with this, be aware that there are New Age practitioners who may adopt spiritual practices from cultures outside of their own, without consent, permission, reciprocity, knowledge, or awareness of how to work with these powerful medicine tools in a good way. These can include the use of smoke, feathers, songs, drums, herbs, and other sacred customs that have often been developed, protected, and passed down by groups of Indigenous wisdom keepers over generations.

It is crucial that we know and honor the context of how these customs made their way to us, and spend time developing a deep understanding of how to engage with medicine work in a way that is reverent, respectful, appropriate, and in right relationship. It is incumbent upon all of us who partake to hold one another accountable, not only for the spiritual hygiene of those who are journeying, but for the cultural heritage of those who continue to experience colonialism as a result of this "psychedelic renaissance." There are often respectful alternatives to customs that are frequently appropriated (Courtney provided the example of using rosemary instead of white sage), and these are worth taking the time to learn.

FOR JOURNEYERS

Especially for those new to psychedelic exploration, there can be a great many questions and curiosities when deciding whether to partake in a journey, and with whom. It is important to have practical guidelines for choosing a facilitator or sitter who is a good fit, as well as to be attuned to one's own intuition and nervous system in order to assess whether a natural ease and trust will be possible. This relationship building is a process that can't be rushed. There needs to be enough space for you as the client to settle into a place of familiarity and trust, and to get comfortable enough to use your voice in the session if needed.

In your process of finding a facilitator and putting a plan in place for a journey, look for someone who embraces your questions and answers them honestly and clearly. For some who hold a more materialist worldview, the notion of spiritual consent may sound far-reaching. However, I have met many people who identify as otherwise nonspiritual, and emerge from psychedelic experiences being wholly convinced of the reality of what they saw, felt, and experienced.

This speaks to the clear need for spiritual preparation for all journeyers. This doesn't have to mean adopting a practice that feels inauthentic or contrived. It can be as simple as setting an intention, lighting a candle, and ensuring that your facilitator is respectful of your worldview and aligned with your preferences around ritual and space holding.

My friends at Fireside Project have created a great resource titled "Questions to Discuss with a Prospective Psychedelic Facilitator."[4] It is readily available online and covers seven major categories of questions, including touch, training, safety planning, and accountability mechanisms. I encourage you to look it up and discuss it with whomever you're considering working with.

FOR FACILITATORS

Establish a consistent process for screening and intake with all of your clients. If the process is too fluid, important steps can be skipped, especially when sitting for a friend or loved one. It is highly important that regardless of the existing level of familiarity, all journeyers are provided adequate preparation.

Know and be very clear about your scope of practice and the skills/ practices you are bringing to the work. How does your scope impact your work? For example, if you are a bodyworker, energy worker, or shamanic practitioner, how do you intend to use or not use these modalities during the session? Be explicit. These need to be discussed and agreed upon ahead of time. If your client is not comfortable with you using certain modalities during the session, be clear on what you can agree to. Honoring their boundaries is essential to acting from a place of consent and doing your part to ensure a positive outcome.

Before the Session

- Take the time to explicitly discuss what consent looks like for each of you.

- Discuss plans for touch, physical space, and any modalities available during the session.

- Put these agreements in writing.

- Go over any standard written documents you use and give ample time (at least several days) for the client to look them over, reflect, and ask questions.

- Have a final check-in before the session and make any needed adjustments to session, safety, and follow-up plans.

During the Session

◆   Honor the agreements that have been made.

◆   Check in regularly.

◆   Take notes of relevant moments, requests, and statements made.

After the Session

◆   Honor agreements regarding check-ins and follow-up care.

◆   Review any notes taken during the session.

◆   Ask for feedback, and create a safe environment for them to provide it.

◆   Make repairs for any missteps.

◆   Discuss expectations and boundaries regarding future interactions.

◆   Consult with community of practice for additional feedback and guidance on any situations you're uncertain about.

IN PRACTICE

I asked Courtney for her views on how we can establish consent with clients and form agreements with them that honor their agency while also creating safety.

> People need to have agency. But we also need to have crisis plans created ahead of time in the event that something does not go right, that still allows that person to have the power of choice. I've definitely had a journey where I was like, "Nope. I want this to end now."

> So, part of informed consent is preparing people that they might have moments where they don't want to continue. And having that conversation so that if something comes up, we have already discussed options for how we can support them. We can rank those interventions in order of their preference and comfort level. We can discuss in what scenarios we would transfer to a hospital, and be transparent about whether that has ever occurred and what those circumstances were. We need to make sure people know their options around crisis planning. Someone might say, "Whatever you do, I don't want you to call the police," and we need to understand why that is important and be clear about whether we can honor that. If you can't, be transparent from the outset so the person can choose whether to work with you or not.

> The responsibility lies on the person facilitating to get serious about their safety planning practices. If a client asks you about a specific risk

management practice and you respond, "Oh, don't worry, I've never had that happen before," that's not sufficient.

Additional Notes

HUMBLE PREPARATION. In the river rafting community, there's this phrase "rigged to flip," which means you tighten and secure all of your gear at all times so it's ready in case the boat flips. You don't only do that when you're about to do something risky. You do it if you're on the water, period. My partner, who had never flipped their raft, was always diligent about this and we never flipped or needed it, but it was a simple way of helping ensure the best possible outcome. I believe that attitude of humility really transfers to our work here. It means knowing that what you're going into is bigger than you and has power beyond you. This enables us to acknowledge that power and create a plan so that we're as ready as we can be for whatever comes up.

FOLLOW-THROUGH. Consent agreements are only as good as their follow-through. This is where trust is deepened and safety is established. The facilitator asks, hears the client, and replies according to the client's response. Without follow-through, agreements made ahead of time can be performative and misleading. During a psychedelic experience, facilitators must be ready to adjust their approach and expectations in real time without defensiveness, negotiating, or taking it personally. This is where inner-work enters the picture—the ability to be aware of and temporarily set aside one's attachments, triggers, needs, and desires for the benefit of the client.

ATTUNEMENT. It's essential that facilitators develop the skill of attunement. Sometimes a "no" or hesitation can be sensed even if it is not verbally stated. For example, the facilitator should not only ask and receive clear consent before touching a client; they should also follow up by asking, "How is this for you?" or "Does this feel helpful?"

Sometimes a client might not have a clear answer readily accessible to them when asked; finding the voice for one's needs and desires is lifelong work, and in altered states, self-doubt, self-awareness, or the desire not to offend can be limiting. In this case deep listening, proactive communication, and attunement to body language and energy systems are important.

The facilitator should have or develop the sensitivity to pick up on subtle nonverbal cues from the client, as well as the flexibility to adjust what they are doing in response. In connection with this, the facilitator needs to practice inviting feedback and creating a welcoming environment for feedback to be offered.

Whenever possible, practice and receive feedback on touch in separate sessions before the psychedelic session. Providing the client an opportunity to practice communicating "yes" and "no" to specific kinds of touch. This can build rapport and ensure there is sufficient communication available between people ahead of psychedelic work.

A NOTE ON INTIMATE PARTNERSHIPS

For those not engaging in a formal facilitator-client dynamic, yet journeying with loved ones such as friends or intimate partners, conversations and agreement around consent will be different, but still of paramount importance. This could be a scenario where a group of people are consuming a substance together, or a situation where one person is journeying and another is the sitter. Many community groups, such as the social circles I was involved with during my experimentation years, have established best practices and rules of thumb for navigating psychedelic experiences within dual relationships.

For example, some couples will journey together but agree not to engage sexually while under the influence. Or friends will journey together but define clear roles and appoint someone to stay sober as the sitter and monitor basic safety considerations during the experience. Within these relationships, boundaries and norms will be different than a formal psychedelic medicine space; however, agreements still need to be made explicit prior to beginning to avoid any unintended consent violations or misunderstandings. In addition to the earlier questions regarding safety planning, here are a few things to discuss, especially with regard to touch:

- What kinds of touch are okay to engage in before, during, and after the experience?

- What are our boundaries around sexual interaction before, during, and after the experience? How is this the same or different from our default agreements?

- How will we communicate about and honor needs and boundaries while under the influence?

- When and how will we debrief the experience and provide and receive feedback?

- How will we address harm if it occurs?

In Conversation with Emma Knighton, LMHC

I spoke with Emma Knighton, LMHC, a leading educator on consent and trauma-informed care in the psychedelic field, about navigating consent. They are someone I have learned a great deal from, and as a friend and colleague, I have witnessed that they truly practice what they preach.

Emma is a white, queer, able-bodied femme with lineage rooted in Celtic Druidry. They have a private practice where they work at the intersection of complex PTSD from childhood abuse, queer identity development, and consciousness exploration. Emma is the Director of Education at Alma Institute, teaches in a variety of other spaces in the psychedelic field, and does organizing work in the psychedelic ecosystem around equity, access, and integrating liberation practices and the spirit of the medicine into organizational strategy and operations. Their clinical, educational, and leadership approach is grounded in queer, consent, feminist, and anti-oppression/pro-liberation theories.

RM: *How would you define consent?*

EK: My definition of consent draws from kink and sex work lineages. In the kink world, I come from a risk-aware consensual kink model that really lines up with trauma-informed care. This means being really aware of the risks that are present, and then moving from that awareness. And then from the sex work community, Betty Martin's work around the Wheel of Consent highly informs everything I do.

The definitions that I use refer to trauma-attuned consent, specifically within psychedelic work. So I define it as the embodied process of cocreating an agreement centered on negotiations of desires, limits, and risk. And then, kind of secondary to that, consent looks at how we grapple with being in relationships while holding the reality that we are all capable of harming each other. And we all have personal and ancestral stories of being harmed living in our bodies.

Consent is a conversation we have; it's a negotiation. But more than that, it's about how our bodies relate to each other. I used to talk about "trauma-informed" consent, and I've changed it to "trauma-attuned" consent. Because informed implies something cognitive, in that you are cognitively aware of someone's trauma history, experience with depression, or medicine work, for example. And when we think about the pretty archaic approaches to informed consent, that is the cultural standard at this point. It's all very cognitive in its approach.

Instead, attunement implies that the body's involved. It implies that you are connecting to your nervous system and someone else's nervous system.

It's acknowledging that these things are factors in how we're able to show up with each other and say, yes, no, or maybe, as we're offering and asking for things.

RM: *When it comes to psychedelic therapy, the idea of expertise is tricky because each person's direct experience with the substance is going to be unique. It can't be standardized, and an outside professional can't really be an "expert" on someone else's journey.*

EK: We have not been trained on how to walk the line of really being immersed in someone's experience while simultaneously maintaining professional boundaries. And that is a ripe place for practitioners' own trauma and shadow to come up. I think that's why we're seeing so many ethical issues right now, this intersection of very different modalities. So the question is: how do I have this deeply intimate, embodied experience with another person where there is a power dynamic present, where I have to be accountable for my own stuff coming up, and I have to go with them on this journey they're on and be responsible for their safety?

Because we're used to polarities, we're used to either coming from a place of a) I'm not even a person in the room, I'm just a blank slate for you to project all your stuff onto, or b) I am fully coming with you. What I love about the consent training I have received outside of this field is the foundational expectation of being connected to the person you're working with while maintaining incredibly clear boundaries. It's a really beautiful framework for how to have these deeply intimate experiences with another body, another human, while staying attuned to your responsibilities, the power differentials that are present, and the myriad influences that are at play.

I really see these frameworks of consent as a way to build culture as a whole, and for how we can live in right relationship with each other. Psychedelics are just one little microcosm of that.

The knowledge of how to live with consent hasn't returned to our bodies yet. And to truly practice consent, we have to be in our bodies. And once you are attuned to that, you can translate it into yes, no, or negotiations.

With trauma, the body's pathway to expressing "yes," "no," or "hey, I need more information" has been disrupted. So we're living with the imprint of events where we've had choice and autonomy taken away from our bodies. Every single person has an experience of being touched when they didn't want to be touched, because babies and children are touched constantly without their consent, because they can't give consent. The developmental stage around two years old is when we start learning consent. Toddlers are just running around saying "no" all the time, and for many people, we have to go back to this stage to unlearn lack of consent and relearn what a consensual relationship with our bodies and other bodies feels like. It's a process of relearning that our bodies actually have this really deep wisdom of what a "yes" feels like, what a "no" feels like, and what that middle ground feels like.

Something that one of my teachers in the Betty Martin lineage says that really sticks with me is that *the degree to which someone can access consent is completely aligned with the degree to which they can access choice in their life.* If you don't have access to choice, because of trauma, history, oppression, disconnection from the body, or anything else, you actually can't consent to things. So that's an important layer to look at: do people truly have options? Do they really feel that they have options? Because without options, there's no consent.

RM: *What are some accessible points for beginning or continuing an embodiment practice that can then help people in their own healing path and their work serving others?*

EK: Well, to start, we have to be in relationship to something else in order to feel our bodies. Our own awareness of ourselves happens in the context of relationships. We can't actually perceive ourselves as separate from anything else without a relational component present. That could be a relationship with your dog, relationship with a tree in your backyard, relationship with the clothes you're wearing. So it begins with the acknowledgment of "other." That actually enables our proprioception and interoception, which are fancy words for being able to feel our bodies.

Taking it slow is super important. If someone says, "Okay, we're gonna get in touch with your body." People will often jump to, "Oh, my God, I'm gonna have to feel really deep emotions, or I'm gonna have to have some kind of intimate touch with another person."

But we can slow it way down. What if you go outside and feel a leaf? Or experience the wind on your skin? Or notice what your favorite sweater feels like? Those sorts of things are easier access points. Going slow enough to find the places of resistance.

The limits that need to be honored are not only the client's, but the facilitator's. And so whatever the outside limit is of the person holding the space, that's as far as the person experiencing the space can go. You can't take anyone further than you've gone yourself. That's part of navigating consent—it's not just the consent of the client, it's important for the facilitators to be incredibly attuned to our own boundaries, capabilities, and limits because those will impact what our clients can experience.

In Conversation with Laura Mae Northrup, MFT

I had the pleasure of speaking with Laura Mae Northrup, MFT, whom I look up to for her grounded, real-world approach to psychedelics.

Laura is a leading voice in the psychedelic field around sexual trauma and healing. She created the Inside Eyes *podcast and is the author of a book that has greatly informed my work, called* Radical Healership: How to Build a Values-Driven Healing Practice in a Profit-Driven World. *She practices somatic and ketamine-assisted psychotherapy and her work focuses on defining sexual violence through a spiritual and politicized lens. I admire Laura for her unflinching and compassionate approach to the messy topics of abuse and healing in and beyond the psychedelic field.*

RM: *Let's get right into the sticky stuff. What comes to mind when we talk about consent within the psychedelic field?*

LMN: First, I think of all the consent violations that have happened. There's certainly a lot of concern within this field based on what's arising around boundary violations with regard to touch, and more specifically, sexual boundary violations and various forms of sexual violence.

When I think about consent in the context of healing, I also think about informed consent. That's something as a therapist that we're supposed to go over and document at the beginning of new therapy relationships.

Within informed consent, what we're doing is defining the boundaries, parameters, and what may occur. To some degree, we're also acknowledging what might occur that's not expected or not ideal. In the psychedelic space, this is huge, because there's a lot of emphasis on the idea that this work is going to heal you rather rapidly. It's going to be "all good, love and light." In actuality . . . you could have a psychotic break. You could come out more suicidal. The guide and journeyer could get into some kind of dynamic together where we're accidentally reenacting the journeyer's trauma. In short, a journeyer could really be struggling after partaking in medicine work.

To have a high capacity for change, there's always going to be a correspondingly intense potential for risk. And that is because the space where profound growth happens only occurs in a very vulnerable context, which means the risk is as high as the potential for gain.

We need to think about someone's capacity to consent. In a dynamic where there's an inherent power imbalance, that's something that has to be thought out. This is especially relevant when you're working with people who are highly traumatized. A lot of trauma involves a consent violation: whether that's physical, sexual, psychological, or emotional abuse. Some kinds of trauma don't involve a consent violation, like a car accident might not involve a consent violation. But most people who have complex PTSD, for instance, who are very drawn to psychedelic medicine (and have been told by the media a thousand times by now that they're going to go get healed by psychedelics) often don't have a healthy relationship with consent due to their previous trauma.

How can we create consent in an environment where people's capacity to consent is wounded? This is where we find higher risk. It's possible that things will happen for people in therapy or in a psychedelic setting that don't necessarily feel supportive. At a later time, a person may feel they didn't actually want an experience that occurred in a medicine session or even a typical therapy session.

One reaction could be, "So, don't do high-risk stuff." However, as I mentioned earlier, high risk comes alongside the high potential for healing. One example in my line of work is people who are very focused on using physical touch in sessions. Many therapists and guides believe that physical touch can be super-healing. But consider if you're working with somebody who has serious trauma. You might do many sessions with them before you even introduce touch or psychedelics. That's the slow kind of exploration that is needed to reduce risk. So, if the client or journeyer is going to have a consent challenge come up where they're unsure about something, this can be navigated early and subtly as opposed to a situation where you took a huge risk with your client.

RM: *Touch and consent are so interlinked, a lot of the places that consent risks or violations show up within psychedelic work have to do with touch. And it's tricky because harm can happen by unwanted touch happening, but also by neglecting to provide touch when it is called for or needed. So it's not as simple as saying that less touch is inherently safer.*

LMN: Something I get asked a lot is, "How can we safeguard against or deal with people who are causing harm in this space?" There's a false assumption in that—and that's the belief that only certain people cause harm. *We need to come to terms with the fact that we all do cause harm and we all have the capacity to cause harm.*

But how do we safeguard? I think something we often miss in this conversation is the question of: how do you become an artist who can make a masterpiece? If someone asked you that, you'd say, well, you paint for twenty years, have a muse, you start out naturally skilled or capable, and so on. And I think people get really confused about what healing practitioners do. *Healing work is an art. Being able to do it and navigate consent, and most of the time not hurt people, is an art.* Not everyone should be doing this work, and that's okay.

I think people need to understand that honing this craft is a commitment that takes years of dedication. I hear people saying, "Oh, I want to do that," but they don't want to go to grad school or do a long training. Which is wild. You want to be an emotional surgeon but you don't want to get training?

If someone wants to be a skilled practitioner, they have to understand they're engaging in a process. I train early career clinicians as they work toward a license and it's so brutal, because most of the time, you're not very good at what you're doing for at least three years. And that's a long time to keep showing up and fumbling through it because you have to practice with real people. I recall being filled with anxiety during that part of my career.

What we can and need to do in any context is create or maintain existing small communities that are working together. So we are in close enough proximity to know about each other's cases because we talk weekly. Regardless of where or how you were trained, it's important to have people close enough to know how we're practicing. We need training, oversight, consultation, community, and a strong expectation that people are doing their own personal work as well. And even with the best protocols, harm still happens.

RM: *When it comes to choosing whom to work with, how can we empower choice and consent when someone wants to work with us and there's already an inherent power dynamic present?*

LMN: It really is an art, and every person holding space should already have done some work and reflection around who is a good person for them to work with and who is not. You should not be working with everyone. This work should happen with the support of a mentor. And related to that, understanding scope of competence, and scope of practice. Scope of practice means: if you're calling me with a medical condition, and I'm not a doctor, that's outside of my scope of practice. With scope of competence, maybe someone is contacting me about an eating disorder and I'm not trained in that. That's a scope of competence issue.

People should be able to articulate very specifically whether they trip-sit or are doing psychedelic therapy. Maybe they can hold a safe container and caring presence, but they will not be offering any psychological support. They need to let folks know that they are not a psychotherapist, and how the work differs. It's really just grounding honestly into what you do, for yourself and your clients. Do I offer a very loving presence? That's not nothing—that's huge. Due to the public narrative, folks are going to think they're getting psychedelic therapy. So we need to be ultra-transparent about the distinctions.

If we're going to use touch in our practice, we always need to be asking, "Why am I touching this person right now? Is it for me? Is it because I'm uncomfortable with what's going on?" And that really extends beyond touch, because there are other ways we can interact in a session that center the practitioner's discomfort rather than the journeyer's.

Watching somebody be on psychedelics is not chill. It can be very activating to witness. They could be making very strange movements. Somebody could be saying strange things; they could be shaking around and speaking in an indecipherable language.

With every intervention, we need to get really curious and honest about why we are making it. With touch, people actually need training. They need to know how and why to touch someone. It's more than my client seems uncomfortable, so I'm gonna hug them. That's not conscious. This person isn't your close friend who's having a hard time. You're holding space for a client. It's different. And often part of healing is actually helping somebody suffer through their process, not soothing them out of it.

RM: *For the facilitator, the work is to be able to track what's happening. This part is different if you're a therapist versus if you're a sitter. Sitters really are learning how to get out of the way while still being present and attentive. It's being attuned, watching and listening for when something's asked to me that I can actually provide support for, and other than that, not intervening in this person's process.*

LMN: There's a lot of downtime. People often decide they want to be a psychedelic guide after they've done a psychedelic. But there's a big difference between being on a psychedelic, which can be very exciting, compared to being with someone who's on a psychedelic, which can be quite boring. People want "action movie therapy"; they want to be there when someone's crying and having a breakthrough.

But in reality, you need to prepare to be a psychedelic guide by thinking of it as an eight-hour meditation retreat. Sometimes, you're just sitting with yourself while somebody is having their process. People need to really spend time thinking about that. It's not necessarily going to be wild and exciting.

Conclusion

Consent work is foundational to both our pain and healing. There is no way to engage with psychedelics without encountering the dynamics of consent, agreements, limits, and risk. When consent is centered, the client has a chance to exercise personal agency, which in itself can be a greatly reparative experience. The person responsible for upholding agreements and protecting client safety is the facilitator. This is power-sharing in action. While the facilitator and client hold two very different roles, partnering in collaboration toward the client's best possible experience renders them as teammates working toward a shared goal or travel companions on an epic quest.

By taking the time to understand the client's intentions and expectations, the facilitator can gauge whether they are a good fit for the client, and when needed, refer out to someone who may be better suited to work with them. The key is reaching and maintaining clarity around each person's roles and responsibilities, and taking the time needed to do this.

CHAPTER 10

Accountability

Defining Accountability

Accountability is a cycle of harm, recognition, and repair. When damage has been done, a reparative healing process needs to take place. Before we can talk about holding one another accountable, it's essential to address the practice of holding ourselves accountable. Taking responsibility for our actions and their impacts can be hard, lifelong work, especially when it hasn't been modeled. It requires us to labor through our own barriers to receiving critique. Only once we get past our own denial, fragility, and excuses can we reach a place where growth can happen. While reconciliation isn't always guaranteed, self-responsibility can at least open the possibility of returning to community after harm has been caused. This long-term repair work rarely happens in isolation—it happens in our homes, partnerships, friendships, professional collaborations, and within the larger movements.

Accountability takes many different forms:

Self-accountability asks each of us to recognize that we live in an interconnected world where our actions have immediate and indirect impacts on our surroundings. We begin by examining our values and belief systems to ensure they are aligned with the needs and well-being of our communities. Then we can cultivate the practice of tracking whether or not our behavior is aligned with these values. But we all have blind spots; this is why we need each other.

Interpersonal accountability can sometimes be enticing. On one hand, there's some primal part of us that feeds off of scandalous news when someone in the community goes rogue. There can be an impulse to see folks who are doing damage taken down; perhaps witnessing these takedowns makes us feel superior. Punishment might create an illusion of safety, or at least, demonstrate that the community has boundaries and agreements we can all lean on. The responsibility here is to ensure that before we expend energy confronting others about their behavior, we check ourselves. We need to ask: "Am I the best person, and is this the best time to call this person in? Is there inner-work that I am responsible for at this moment? And importantly, am I ready to participate in an accountability process without doing further damage?"

Institutional accountability is the elusive fantasy we can't seem to get enough of. In the psychedelic space, observers often point to major corporations, or "corporadelics," as the demise of this emerging field, and many of us join in by expressing our outrage on comment threads and podcasts. Perhaps this is because it is easy to see large corporations as faceless monsters to rail against. But again, we have to go deeper. Who is leading these organizations? What worldviews and assumptions are they operating under, and what wounds or fears might be beneath behaviors we see as problematic? Importantly, what are the parts of ourselves being uncomfortably reflected in their behaviors? How might we be embodying problematic qualities in our own lives and practices?

Accountability becomes a long-term process of choosing to stay in relationship when it is safe to do so. We set out to do this while understanding that as flawed humans, we will certainly hurt one another. This is why we need clear agreements, boundaries, safety parameters, and systems for repair. While it isn't always safe or possible to stay in connection with people who have done harm, there is a spectrum of ways to deal with harm that are proportionate, humane, and within our capacity as individuals and organizations. I believe this added effort can create more opportunity for long-term healing than the scorched-earth options our society validates.

Exploring Accountability

For many years, the global psychedelic community has weathered difficult ruptures as patterns of problematic behavior have come to light. While calls for accountability have been increasing, we have very few frameworks or collectives that can meaningfully support it in practice. Such are the challenges of a decentralized, citizen-powered movement: it is as diverse and situational as the psychedelic experience itself, and accountability is not a one-size-fits-all process. The ways we approach massive, powerful institutions often look very different from the ways we approach those in our immediate social groups or those in broader communities. Additionally, creating new systems takes a lot of resources, people power, and knowledge.

It has been established that the psychedelic space has an abuse problem. We have seen sexual assault in underground healing environments, and leaders aligning with sexual predators. We've witnessed the shameless commodification of ceremonial practices and the silencing of voices championing equity and diversity. More issues are bound to surface as we attempt to create practical systems for accountability that can keep up with this rapid expansion.

How do we address these issues? Community accountability and transformative justice frameworks can help guide us.

The mainstream paradigm of accountability is rooted in the legal system. It is centered around the concept of penalty. Simply put, this means that if someone breaks the law or a societal contract, they will be punished, often by removal or being made to experience the same pain and suffering they have caused. In this context, justice is a contract between the individual and the state, and harm is defined by legal institutions. It can be static, rigid, and lacking in nuance. Among the many issues with this punitive model is the simple fact that the needs and experiences of survivors and those impacted are often an afterthought. In addition, carceral culture does little to prevent further harm, rehabilitate the person responsible, or address the underlying conditions that contributed to the event.

If we don't dedicate ourselves to practicing new ways to intervene on harm while the psychedelic movement is still relatively small, the fallout could be much greater. We could overlook major harms occurring around us because we don't feel equipped to address them, or we could replicate the racist, classist power structures that shape the legal concept of accountability. If we want to be a culture built on the cornerstones of healing and relationship, we will need to find ways to embody these values in our approaches to accountability.

THE OPPORTUNITY

There is no singular formula for addressing harm and conflict; the needs of each community and context are unique. That's why these conversations need to be taking place from our smallest pods of community to our largest public forums. We need to define explicit yet adaptable agreements so we can put them into practice at home. Whatever we create together in the microcosm will ultimately determine what takes shape on a larger scale.

In the past few years, I have been brought into *many* behind-the-scenes conversations where I have been earnestly warned about problematic individuals and organizations in the psychedelic scene. I have been given firsthand accounts of behaviors ranging from ethically questionable to outright violent and predatory.

Perhaps this secretive dynamic is a reflection of the established contract around psychedelics. While the space is splintered, I believe we share at least one cause—to destigmatize and create safer access to psychedelics—and thus, we feel the responsibility to look out for one another. This is a network of people who understand the potential legal and reputational ramifications of outing anyone who is a part of the psychedelic underground. *But are we more loyal to the movement for psychedelic access itself than to the people who have been harmed within it?*

Over and over, when I hear these cautionary tales, the same questions arise for me:

Have these concerns been brought to the person in question? Is mycelial, grapevine-style dialogue the best way to establish safety amongst ourselves? How can we move forward in ways that actually interrupt patterns of harm while promoting repair? I fear that the current nonconfrontational approach allows problematic behavior to continue, not only due to the shroud of secrecy caused by prohibition but also because of our own unwillingness, on an interpersonal level, to address it head-on.

Those who are informed of ethical violations have to contend with how to respond. I have been in situations where I wondered:

What is my role in addressing this situation? What do I have the capacity for?

Should I caution the people around me?

Should I speak with the accused person directly?

How do we get to the truth of a situation, and at what point should these truths be made public? Who gets to decide?

When should someone be muted, removed from a position of leadership, or barred from participating in community?

How do we set terms for their reentry?

ACCOUNTABILITY IN THE WORLD

Ultimately, the nature of accountability is relational. The act of uncovering messy truths and the challenging processes of responsibility often happen at kitchen tables and park benches, not boardrooms and convention stages.

Fortunately, we don't have to reinvent the wheel. The psychedelic community may be new to the justice discussion, but leaders from other disciplines have spent many years engaging with the messy, daily practice of addressing and repairing harm. We would be wise to learn from these leaders. If we do, the psychedelic field will be better off for it.

THE TRANSFORMATIVE JUSTICE APPROACH

When we reimagine the idea of safety within community, there are two terms that are often used interchangeably: *restorative justice* and *transformative justice*. While they are related, they have key differences.

The United Nations Working Group on *Restorative Justice (RJ)* defines it this way: "A process whereby parties with a stake in a particular offense resolve collectively how to deal with the aftermath of the offense and its implications for the future. In essence, we seek to repair the harms caused by crime and violence."

The process seeks to restore the conditions that were present before harm took place. RJ efforts often work in tandem with local judicial systems.

Transformative Justice (TJ) goes even deeper. It seeks to address the context in which harms occurred and, through a community-centered approach, catalyze long-term shifts in the very fabric of society. This can serve not only to prevent harm, but also to create conditions that lead to healing and thriving.

For years, transformative justice efforts have been a part of the movement toward building healthier, more intact communities and reducing the reliance on policing as our only means of creating safety. It is a holistic approach that first focuses on resourcing the victims/survivors of harm, who are often erased within the punitive justice system. Rehabilitating the person responsible is a secondary consideration, in the spirit of prevention. In addition, it holds an eye toward the source and root cause of the harm, rather than treating individual situations as isolated incidents. This enables us to make systematic shifts that can ultimately ripple outward and help reshape the culture of our communities as a whole.

Transformative justice understands that the harms we inflict upon one another are the downstream effects of larger dysfunctions within our society. They may stem from a culture shaped by scarcity, disconnection, domination, and intergenerational trauma. In order to truly prevent harm from repeating, we have to transform the underlying issues and the belief structures that uphold them.

Interrogating our community standards and assumptions, strengthening interdependence, and addressing the root causes of harm are at the heart of transformative justice.

Benefits of Transformative Justice

- It enables intervention before small harms and patterns escalate into major problems.
- It centers the needs and experiences of survivors or those impacted.
- It enables all involved to increase their capacity for clear communication, generative conflict, and ownership of responsibility.
- It creates an opportunity for the person who has done harm to reflect on and understand the impact of their actions.
- It requires an actionable plan for repair.
- It cultivates greater safety, resilience, and trust within the community.

Limitations of Transformative Justice

- Accountability processes sometimes happen months or years after an incident has occurred.

- Defining repair is much harder when death or major harm has occurred.
- Results are slower and more systemic (we have to be invested in the long view).
- Confrontation can be extremely uncomfortable.
- Those who are confronted cannot be coerced into accountability processes.
- Making amends doesn't often have a clear timeline or resolution.
- Community involvement over time is required.

Potential Misuse of Transformative Justice

- People who aren't committed to their inner-work might harness the language or tools of accountability in an attempt to control situations or deflect culpability.
- People might repeat serious harms over time and rely on the optics of transformative justice to save face when held accountable.
- Those invested in upholding existing power structures might discourage efforts toward transformative justice, as it is rooted in systemic change.

WHAT IF WE ARE ALL RESPONSIBLE?

There is a tempting, self-righteous satisfaction in punishing or doing away with people we view as problematic. Part of the reason punitive systems exist within our society is that they allow us to rely on a convenient binary. When we frame complex situations as right/wrong, good/bad, or involved/not involved, we get a free pass to look the other way. We get to be the heroes or innocent bystanders (until it is our turn to be the villains, that is). Effectively, we participate in a fantasy in which we absolve ourselves of the nuanced and laborious process of conflict transformation.

Community-based approaches to accountability can have major benefits, but they require a lot of work. If the goal of accountability is to interrupt cycles of harm and create vitality in our communities, we must also work to create healthier systems at the root level. This reimagining takes all of us. In an interview with the Barnard Center for Research on Women, Esteban Kelly, cofounder of AORTA (Anti-Oppression Resource & Training Alliance),[1] put it this way:

> [Transformative justice] distributes culpability a bit. Which isn't to say it is even, but everyone holds some amount. What environment enabled the silencing to go on, such that this pattern was able to continue until a crisis? What allowed things to escalate? What were the subtle hints

around male supremacy, sexism, white supremacy, or different forms of class power that gave people hidden messages that this was acceptable or that we're not going to intervene?[2]

STEPS OF ACCOUNTABILITY IN TRANSFORMATIVE JUSTICE

Transformative justice acknowledges that there are no quick fixes to complex problems. Calling someone in is a first step, but there is no way of knowing how they will respond. Given the complex dynamics that can often lead to damaging behavior, it is possible that someone will refuse to participate in peacemaking efforts. If they are willing, however, a loose framework can look this way:

1. **Identifying the harm:** A problematic behavior or pattern is identified— by the individual, someone affected, or the surrounding community.

2. **Calling in:** The person in question is called in. If you are called in, it can take some time to wade through your initial reaction and emotional activation, but ultimately, see if you can receive the call to accountability as a loving act. You are being invited to change a behavior instead of being exiled because of it.

3. **Taking responsibility:** Feeling bad or saying sorry isn't enough here. We need to own our part. True accountability requires that we take responsibility for our actions and identify where we had freedom of choice when we may have felt we had no options. *This also requires that we take the time to notice patterns of behavior and identify what new behaviors need to be learned in order to prevent repeating the harm in the future.*

4. **Commitment to repair:** The person responsible dedicates themself to repairing the harms that were caused and communicates this to harmed parties.

5. **Clarifying agreements and actionable steps:** Ideally, those impacted will be involved in the decision-making process around what repair should look like. The more specific you can be, the better. For example, if the person responsible is in a position of leadership, do they need to be asked to step down from their platform for a set period of time? If someone has harmed another person in the community directly, do they need to help cover the cost of healing services?

6. **Following up and ongoing relationship:** This is where the rubber meets the road. Change takes time, and the process is not linear. To fulfill agreements and develop new habits, people need to be held in community, while

also keeping those who have been harmed safe. Follow through on commitments made, and lean on trusted peers who can keep you accountable.

Sometimes, harm is so deep and shattering that basic steps toward repair may seem simplistic. For example, what if someone dies during an underground medicine retreat or a clinical trial? Worse, what if there are efforts to conceal or rewrite the narrative of what has happened? When facing situations where the loss of life has occurred, the family of the deceased must be heard and empowered to define what efforts toward repair feel supportive on their own terms.

But what if the person in question refuses to accept responsibility? What if the survivor or person impacted has no interest in being a part of an accountability process? Can transformative justice principles still serve when the process is less tidy?

I spoke with Esteban Kelly about his perspectives on creating a culture of accountability within movements. In addition to being a cofounder and worker-owner of AORTA Co-op, he also spent fifteen years as a volunteer member of Philly Stands Up, a community-based transformative justice collective that worked directly with people who caused harm in sexual assault situations. Through PSU, Kelly amplified the lessons of transformative justice to help local communities navigate scenarios of interpersonal harm and healing. He said:

> If someone won't be accountable, we are not going to do something coercive, contribute to call-out culture, or publicly shame them. We ask survivors, please don't do a public take-down of this person; we're not calling to cancel people. Instead, we might suggest that communities mute them or say they should not be platformed, but we ultimately want to draw people back into networks of trust. When possible, we want to direct resources and coaching to them so they are more capable of the change those around them know they need.

Developing Muscle Memory in the Accountability Process

Accountability is a process, not an endpoint we arrive at. It requires acknowledging and taking responsibility for the harm that's been caused, making amends however possible, and taking steps to change behavior so the harm does not continue. This requires that we develop skills in introspection, communication, and sitting with discomfort. It requires us to ask, "What are the actions I can take to make things as right as possible, given that I can't go back and undo what was done?"

Theoretically, these practices could transfer seamlessly into the psychedelic community. Is this a utopian vision, or is there hope for a lasting, truly just psychedelic movement that doesn't self-destruct during its ascent? That depends on how committed we are to the process of change, first within ourselves and our immediate circles. Kelly offers up the long view:

> This rhythm of theory, action, and reflection has to be iterative and constantly evolving. What are we trying to do at a societal level if we can't even figure it out in our own communities? These small exercises are maps and instructions for how we can reprogram things at a larger scale.
>
> Transformative justice doesn't really make sense until you are involved in testing it out and applying it in the laboratory of your life. Testing it out in low-stakes situations will help these concepts make sense. Then, when the going gets tough, you have the muscle memory to handle more difficult scenarios.
>
> There's a certain role that everyday facilitators and community organizers can play. Right now, that is where the gap is. So, how can we rise to the occasion ourselves to take these skills that seem professionalized and translate them into everyday skills? Transformative justice is not about running social services through nonprofits and institutions. Those may be effective for other things, but there's something else that can happen in a less codified way, in these intimate TJ settings, and that's the change we're trying to achieve.

In other words, change begins at home. We've got to redefine justice on a personal level and learn to be accountable for ourselves and our immediate circles before we're ready to make institutional change. Here are a few places to start:

For All of Us

1. Invite mentors and elders into your life.
2. Commit to a practice of brutally honest personal reflection.
3. Get in touch with your body. Notice what comes up when you feel guilty, ashamed, threatened, accused, or misunderstood. Practice noticing these emotions in minor situations and develop tools for managing them.
4. Practice rupture and repair cycles in personal relationships.
5. Learn how to apologize effectively.
6. Develop capacity for uncomfortable conversations.
7. Ask your peers for feedback.
8. Create a culture of radical honesty and authenticity in your relationships.
9. Practice following through on your commitments.
10. Enlist a specific set of trusted "tough love" peers to be in close proximity and call you in when needed.

How do we choose the right people to be our inner circle of accountability? Esteban Kelly lays out some considerations.

> It might not be your best friend. It might be your coworker, sibling, or neighbor. It's more about the quality of the relationship than the quantity of people. Who do you share a depth of trust with? Where are the spaces in your life where you can receive direct feedback? The broken conditions of the world can feed into our ideas of victimization and defensiveness.

> When you're activated, you may not be able to really hear critique. Who can, despite this, hang in there through the worst of the hurdles you put up, have compassion for your human experience, and essentially bear-hug you into accountability? Who can say: "Yes, you can scream, cry, yell, etc. I'm able to hear your initial round of deflection and excuses. I may or may not validate them. But now that that's off your chest, can you get to a place where you're able to listen? It may be weeks or months later, but I'll be here as a support person."

For Journeyers

While adverse events are rare, it's important to know that they can stem not only from the substance itself, but also from the actions of a poorly trained or unethical facilitator. Spend time understanding what you can expect from your facilitator, especially when you are working with a new person or new substance.

Ask your facilitator the following questions:

- What community support do you have in place to keep you accountable for your actions?

- What recourse is there if an incident happens within our session?

- Have you ever had a rupture or breach of ethics with a previous client?

- If so, can you tell me about what happened and how it was handled? What is your relationship with that person like now?

If your facilitator is unable or unwilling to answer these questions, it's a signal to move on and find someone else who can.

For Facilitators

This entire chapter is for you. Spend time sitting with any sticking points that came up while you were reading. Identify two or three people in your life whom you can trust to have hard conversations with you. This could be a mentor, elder, coworker, or another trusted individual. Ask them if they will be available to you for accountability in your work as a facilitator. Spend some time discussing your unique ethical vulnerabilities and laying out strategies for safeguarding against them. Form agreements around how you will keep them informed of your process, and how they can approach you if they notice something that needs attention.

Spend some time reflecting on your personal relationship to accountability and punishment.

- What were you taught growing up about justice and responsibility?
- Whom did you receive these messages from?
- What happens within you when you make a choice that is out of alignment with your ethics?
- How do you respond when someone offers you feedback or calls you in to an accountability process?
- What examples do you have of times you have navigated this?

Read over the section for journeyers and spend some time preparing for the questions listed there.

In Conversation with Leia Friedwoman

I was a fan of Leia from a distance for quite some time. We finally met during a workshop she organized in 2022 for leaders in the psychedelic field, to train with Kai Cheng Thom under her "Loving Justice" framework. This was the first time I had been in a setting where we could unpack these important strategies for conflict management alongside peers who understood the nuances of psychedelic work.

Leia Friedwoman, MS, loves to connect the dots as a teacher, writer, and agent of healing. She earned her master's degree in clinical psychology in 2013 and worked as an in-home therapist before psychedelics turned her world inside out. Today, Leia approaches healing work through a lens of social and environmental justice, utilizing trauma-informed, somatic, relational, and developmental frameworks to support people on their journey toward more felt wholeness and connection. She is deeply grateful for the opportunity to study and practice accountability and transformative justice in her community. Leia hosts a podcast called The Psychedologist: *"consciousness positive radio."*[3]

In a *Lucid News* article, "How the Psychedelic Community Should Respond to Sexual Abuse," Leia writes:

In the aftermath of abuse, there are questions and considerations for survivors, therapists, community members to take into account; this is not just a problem for people who have been abused to solve. Survivors may fear coming out to others about what happened to them. They may face victim blaming, gaslighting, or denial that the therapists they work with are capable of abuse. Survivors of abuse may even be threatened with legal action for defamation. In addition, those who want to confront their abusers may feel conflicted about having been hurt by a person who they looked up to or placed trust in.

In spite of this, telling one's story can also be a liberating and empowering action, one that may encourage others to come out and seek support, breaking the silence on psychedelic therapy abuse.[4]

RM: *How did you become interested in this sort of subset of the work, which is really supporting survivors and facing some of the less glamorized parts of psychedelic healing and its underbelly?*

LF: While my heart lies at the preventative end of violence, supporting survivors feels like the most important thing that I could do in this moment, as someone who's been touched by these medicines, works in this space, and carries her own experience of sexual assault prior to her first psychedelic ceremony.

I know that it's easy for people to fall through the cracks. I'm always learning about how I can better show up to support folks who have been harmed in the context of psychedelic sessions. I'm not an expert at this, and probably never will be. It has been a big learning journey for me to recognize and responsibly hold the power that I have as a figure in the psychedelic arena and an organizer of these survivor spaces.

RM: *What do you see as the role of witnesses and community members in these instances of harm?*

LF: I think something often missed in this conversation is that the psychedelic world is not special or distinct. These same abuses of power happen in traditional therapy, in religious and spiritual communities, in kink and BDSM spaces, and within families. That's sad and horrifying, and also it gives us the opportunity to learn from how other communities have handled abuses of power.

Kai Cheng Thom has taught me that when we are in or near a conflict, we will probably be experiencing internal conflict as well. How we relate to that internal conflict will have some bearing on how we show up to support the harmed party, call the person who caused harm into accountability or pursue changes to the structures and systems that gave rise to the harm happening in the first place.

After harm, everyone needs systems of support. To anyone who finds themselves inside or on the outskirts of conflict, I tell them to ask themselves, who can I process this with? How will I know if it's getting to be too much for me? How will I know when I need to push myself a little bit more to go to that edge of my comfort in this situation? If there's an urge to rush, can I slow down? Is there something I'm being asked to do? What does my conscience say is right? I highly recommend Mia Mingus's work on Pod Mapping for this.

In the "Loving Justice" workshop series, Kai Cheng taught about how we can escalate or deescalate a conflict. In the case of an abuse of power, it's important to escalate and ensure that no more harm happens. This could look like removing a practitioner who has caused harm from their position of power so that no one else is harmed.

We should examine our own biases, such as attachment relationships. If someone I love gets called into an accountability process, I'll need to check myself and own that my perspective on the situation cannot be objective. I may be subject to delusions, [thinking] because I love this person and they've never hurt me, it's impossible that they could actually hurt someone else.

It is not loving to enable someone to continue harming others or to idly watch them not face their issues. bell hooks talks about how love, which has the power to transform us, requires dedicated work. Something I've learned from supporting survivors is that bystanders can create just as much harm and disconnection as the person who was abusive. I have been a bystander before, and I regret that.

If someone I love gets called in/out, I may be able to support their process of accountability because they trust me and know that I won't stop loving them, even if they reveal some more shadowy sides or they admit to doing something that hurt another person. I'm deeply grateful to the people who still loved and supported me, even as I showed sides of myself that I was ashamed of.

I would like to see more people getting interested in studying and practicing restorative and transformative justice in psychedelic communities. I'm so honored that Kai Cheng Thom has been willing to step into some of our psychedelic spaces with these teachings, and I hope that more groups will feel inspired to invite the many wonderful teachers and practitioners of RJ and TJ to empower us in preventing and facing harm when it happens. It is important that we pay these teachers generously for their important work, and especially that we recognize we are borrowing the resource of their expertise for a time during which they are not available to their own communities. This is a gift, which I would compare to the curanderos who leave their people to come and facilitate ayahuasca ceremonies for Westerners.

I have learned these perspectives from the survivors, my teachers, the Creative Interventions toolkit, and time spent in reflection, and sitting with myself and in community. I am not an expert on these topics, I make mistakes.

I hope to always be learning about how to better prevent harm and support survivors. I hope to get better at asking myself the right questions and sitting with the difficult or elusive answers.

With that caveat, in my view, I think the community should try to find out what the survivors/harmed party(s) are asking for and what can be done to support them. The community might be able to come together to raise funds; maybe the survivor wants to get out of town and stay in an Airbnb elsewhere or travel to stay with loved ones. Maybe they need funds for therapy, food, or transportation. Maybe they just want you to listen to them. They may need or want something that isn't possible for them to get at this time. Can you hold space for them through that as well?

If you find yourself in a close relationship with a person who caused harm, they may need help understanding the difference between intention and impact. Two resources I recommend are a document titled "How Do You Process Uncomfortable Information?" by the Centre for Holding Space,[5] and the Philly Stands Up Accountability Roadmap.[6] I also love AccountabilityMapping.com for coaching support. And Rebecca, *you* wrote a great article for *Psychedelics Today*[7] about a roadmap to accountability in psychedelic communities!

What I would say to someone being accused of harm is that there may have been events in your past or in your lineage that you have not fully under-stood and sorted out, resulting in you harming someone else. You may not have understood that what you were doing was harmful. Try to look at this experience as an opportunity for you to do the necessary learning, healing, and repair so that you don't do something like this again. It may be that you need to shift the sort of work you do and not work directly with vulnerable clients anymore. I believe that your accountability will be, most of all, liber-ating for *yourSelf*. You are worth taking this journey.

RM: *I wonder if you have any thoughts on the critiques of transformative justice, as well as the merits. How do you sit with those tensions?*

LF: This isn't a critique, but maybe a point of clarification: *taking someone out of a position of power is not a punishment. It's a safety measure.* You can do trans-formative justice and also remove someone from the role they have abused or are abusing. I've seen people in positions of power say that they're getting punished when they lose their position. That's not punishment; it's safety.

Importantly, it is on all of us to critically engage our deepest parts and investigate whether we want to punish people. It's a valid desire, and I think most of us can relate to wanting someone who hurt us to be punished. Let us bring those impulses out of the shadows so that they won't covertly be impacting our decisions.

I think one mistake that can happen is sometimes these processes give a lot of attention and resources to the people who caused harm. If they weren't ready to be accountable, then you can't get that resource back. I believe it should be really clear that someone wants to be accountable before a lot of resources are invested in them. Those resources could go to supporting the healing of the harmed party(s), and/or go into community coming together to transform the conditions that gave rise to that particular harm.

My sense is that many of the critiques of TJ indicate a lack of understanding of the framework. For example, some people say that transformative justice enables abusers to perform feeling sorry and make shallow repairs that don't actually fix the problem in the first place, meanwhile further traumatizing the harmed parties. While I don't doubt that this can sometimes be the case, especially with high-profile cases of harm, it does not mean that transformative justice doesn't work, or even that that process failed. Mariame Kaba and Shira Hassan say in *Fumbling Towards Repair*[8] that there is something to be gained from every process, and that to classify it as a success or a failure limits the potential of learning from these experiences.

There's something else I wanted to bring up. Transformative justice work has parallels to psychedelics. The oldest of these traditions comes from Indigenous communities. And now, there are people who have been raised outside of an Indigenous context in a capitalistic colonialist context, who are working with these modalities, these medicines, and there are pitfalls to that. With transformative justice, these technologies arose out of communities that handled everything from within. In many cases, they could not go to the police without engaging even more risk. The technologies of TJ and RJ have come out of queer, disabled, BIPOC communities. So when I see the modality being taken out of its context, I think that we need more elders and more teachers to be part of this process with us, so it doesn't get co-opted to be something else entirely.

Just as with psychedelics, there will be new modalities and traditions that arise. But we could listen to what the elders have said and are saying. Because they are the ones who've been through the learning processes and deserve the resources to teach and help support this knowledge to grow in our field. I'm a huge proponent of going outside of the psychedelic community to bring in teachers.

This is a really weird space to be practicing accountability, because people are not only in community together, people are also getting paid; it's people's jobs. So there's a lot on the line. Whereas in a social group, when there's a transgression, or a rupture, and someone could not be accountable, maybe they lose some friends. Or they show up and make a meaningful repair, and they still get to have their friends. In this field, being called out also threatens people's livelihoods. I think it feels like they have more to lose. But if "do no harm" is their ethic, then it's actually much riskier to continue practicing without exploring your accountability. More importantly, it really sucks to screw up your job, but nothing is worse than screwing up someone's life and health, especially someone who came to you for *help*.

That's why I appreciate the framing around consequence culture, which is often incorrectly described as canceling people. It's more of consequences such as deplatforming or requiring changes before supporting someone. We're not coming out here with pitchforks and wanting to condemn anyone. That doesn't help us.

One very important thing at the heart of all this is we have to listen to survivors. This doesn't just have to be psychedelic survivors. For any person with lived experience of survivorship, we need to have their perspectives inform this growing movement.

In Conversation with Juliana Mulligan

Juliana Mulligan is a trusted person I look to for guidance and solidarity. She has firsthand experience navigating accountability and repair processes in the ibogaine field, and she brings a great deal of heart and critical analysis to her work. In addition to her direct lived experience as a patient and her work guiding best practices in ibogaine clinics, she is also a board member at Alma Institute and coauthored the Fireside Project articles "Warning Signs When Selecting a Psychedelic Facilitator" and "Questions to Discuss with a Prospective Psychedelic Facilitator."[9] These are hugely valuable resources that I encourage everyone to check out and share with newcomers to the field.

Juliana Mulligan is a formerly opioid-dependent person, formerly incarcerated, and has been a working member of the ibogaine treatment community for ten years. In 2011, with the help of ibogaine treatment, Juliana left opioids behind and set off on a path to transform the way drug users and their treatment are approached. As of this writing, she is soon to complete her Master of Social Work at NYU and is the Psychedelic Program Coordinator at the Center for Optimal Living. She also runs Inner Vision Ibogaine, which supports people in preparation and integration around ibogaine treatment. She has worked in multiple ibogaine clinics, presented at various psychedelic and harm-reduction conferences, and is the author of the "Guide to Finding a Safe Ibogaine Clinic."[10] She has taught about ibogaine at Charité University in Berlin and Southwestern College in New Mexico, and has written for multiple publications about ibogaine, including Double Blind magazine and Chacruna.

RM: *How did this two-part project, with Fireside Project: Warning Signs and Questions to Discuss with Facilitators, occur?*

JM: Joshua White and I were talking about the ongoing issues in the field and discussing different situations we were each dealing with. And I think the need for this type of resource just kind of came up organically in conversation. We started going back and forth with items we felt were important to have on the list and eventually landed on this final version.

The problem is that psychedelics are getting sold as this panacea, and this magical fix, and as this thing that just automatically will make people better humans, which is not true, but that's the hype that's being projected around it. There are many people coming into this space thinking, "Oh, well, this is a healing community, I can totally trust these people if they're facilitating a psychedelic ceremony or treatment." But the thing is that psychedelics can enhance any quality in a person, including narcissistic tendencies, for example.

Often people are not aware that, because a lot of this work is happening in legal gray areas or in the underground, there is no one to report anything to and no way to ask for help. There's no supervision. There's no oversight. There's no community of accountability for a lot of this work that's happening. People don't know that they're walking into an unmonitored space where there are often no safety protocols being enforced. So it's really hard to choose a facilitator when you're coming in new to the community and you don't know about these issues. That's why we felt like this guide is important, to break down what to look for.

RM: *The growth of this field has really outpaced public education and culture building. We haven't broadly established cultural norms within the psychedelic field, because it's emerging out of the shadows and because Indigenous tradition has largely been erased.*

JM: There's not a thorough understanding of interpersonal dynamics, such as personal responsibility and how to take accountability when there's harm in this community. There are many ongoing conflicts between individuals that are never properly addressed or resolved. Generally speaking, most people are terrified of punishment. And often people equate accountability with punishment and shame.

And so in my experience, when I've tried to approach someone and say, "Hey, I felt like this harm happened, can we look at it?" Regardless of how I've approached them, some have immediately jumped into denial, gaslighting, or defensiveness. Our culture has taught us to avoid accountability since we were children, because to admit to wrongdoing is to be punished and shamed. We live in a punishment-based society, so even in this field, we have people largely still working from that old-school, violent, Judeo-Christian punishment mindset. So people are desperate not to make mistakes and they can't tolerate the feeling when they do. Which, we all do make mistakes.

Right now we need to relearn how to exist in healthy communities and how to be vulnerable. Many people don't know how to do that because our society, under patriarchy, tells us that being vulnerable is a weakness; in reality, it's the bravest thing anybody can do.

RM: *Vulnerability also seems more possible within a container of some sort of existing relationship. We can expose our flaws when there is trust and goodwill established. It's a step often skipped in our workplaces and collaborations; then when conflicts erupt, things become very cold, calculating, and transactional.*

JM: I believe most people in this society have often unconscious deep-rooted abandonment issues because we have been abandoned by society. This society does not support talking about what we feel, and feeling is at the heart of being human. Our families can reinforce the ethos of this society. It makes sense that accountability could feel like a threat of being abandoned again—because you've made a mistake, they're going to leave you.

Living in a society that doesn't teach you how to live with feelings creates a huge wound. Modern psychology talks about abandonment issues, but it talks about it on an interpersonal level. Let's talk about it on a societal grand level—it's the system that's creating this initial abandonment.

I've heard some dismiss the transformative justice model after witnessing a process that didn't go as hoped. But there's a spectrum of how a process like that could work and there needs to be room for flexibility. Structures have to be able to be adapted per situation, and sometimes if something doesn't work, there just needs to be some tweaks. There isn't one right way to do things, and when people become so attached to the "right" way that they become threatened by other ways of working or being—this is dangerous.

With psychedelic therapy, we're often working with people who are coming to us from a very vulnerable place. Often folks are working on major traumas. You don't know what's going to happen—you're giving them a super-powerful medicine that might rip open their psyche. It's a lot to carry as a single person. And because our society is hyper-individualistic, people try to carry that as a single person and they get burned out, and then that's when dangerous things start to happen.

I believe a lot of the scenarios that have gone wrong could have been avoided if there was more community collaboration and if there was a supervision process. Specifically, with ibogaine treatment, we need to have supervision groups or supervisors checking in with people about what's going on. If we could have a community supervision process that was supportive, and not about punishment, I think that would make a major difference.

RM: *Are there lessons you've learned, or things you've seen people learn, that you're hoping will make it into best practices for the field generally?*

JM: We need more support for the facilitators who are doing this important work—therapy, retreats, and networks of care for personal crises. There needs to be a structure, and funding for that structure, that would support facilitators in taking care of themselves and taking breaks if needed.

I think those of us working as providers also really need to take the time to understand the limitations of what we can provide for people. There's a lot of this thing I call psychedelic heroism: this idea that serving people medicine is going to save people or instantly heal them. That's not a thing—as providers, what we're doing is creating a container for people to rediscover their own power; we aren't bestowing onto them something that they didn't already have. We need to do away with this popular hero shaman archetype. Yes, there are real shamans, but us folks from colonizing countries need to be extremely careful about placing ourselves on pedestals. It just reinforces a hierarchy and sets up a very unhealthy and uneven power dynamic that is ripe for harm.

RM: *What do you think are good things to aspire to, and what does success in this field look like?*

JM: I think people should aspire to increase accessibility, to create systems that are more collaborative and community-based, rather than one person at the top. I think that we should value uplifting the Indigenous traditions where these medicines come from; we should prioritize and be proud when these people's voices are centered and included in every initiative. It's time to stop worshiping the pursuit of patents, FDA approval, having our names on research papers, and being traded on the stock market. These are colonial values. To me, the marker of success? Safety, accessibility, and true reciprocity.

Conclusion

The theory of transformation is one thing; the embodied, lived experience of it is something else entirely. As many of us can attest, the cosmic downloads we receive during a psychedelic experience might be profound, but the real magic happens as we integrate these insights into our lives. The same is true for accountability: documentaries, books, and philosophies of change are solid starting points, but they carry with them a call to integrate this knowledge meaningfully into our daily lives. Otherwise, it's just theory.

Alignment and integrity begin within ourselves and expand into our relationships, our networks, and perhaps ultimately, even global coalitions. Just as raindrops fill a stream, streams feed into rivers, and rivers become the ocean, it's impossible to separate the individual from the collective. We should not underestimate the value of ground-level practice, especially with such expansive ideas.

The topic of accountability can be charged. Many of us have had experiences where harm was not properly addressed, or where punishments were heavy-handed, reactionary, or did not take time to hear the people who were impacted. While the work of accountability is messy, imperfect, and asks for community participation, we can find ways to address problems without perpetuating violence.

We have an opportunity to set the tone and shape the culture of this work by how we conduct ourselves, cultivate community, and organize our institutions and advocacy efforts. By modeling and upholding clear, compassionate systems for accountability, bringing our best selves to our interactions, and following through when issues need to be addressed, I believe we can prevent the invasive seedlings of harm from growing into weeds that choke out the beautiful potential of this field.

CHAPTER 11

History

You want to know what this [war on drugs] was really all about? The Nixon campaign in 1968, and the Nixon White House after that, had two enemies: the antiwar left and Black people. You understand what I'm saying?

We knew we couldn't make it illegal to be either against the war or Black, but by getting the public to associate the hippies with marijuana and Blacks with heroin, and then criminalizing both heavily, we could disrupt those communities. We could arrest their leaders, raid their homes, break up their meetings, and vilify them night after night on the evening news.

Did we know we were lying about the drugs? Of course, we did.

—JOHN EHRLICHMAN, Assistant to the President for
Domestic Affairs under President Richard Nixon

Approaching History

IMPORTANT NOTES

Authorship: This chapter and the following chapter, 12, titled "Reciprocity," are coauthored with my esteemed colleague, Juliette Mohr. Juliette (she/her) is a woman of Filipino, Irish, and Portuguese ancestry living in California's East Bay. She has been professionally involved in the psychedelic space since 2019, previously affiliated with organizations such as Students for Sensible Drug Policy (SSDP), Intercollegiate Psychedelics Network (IPN), HowToUsePsychedelics.com (HTUP), Multidisciplinary Association for Psychedelic Studies Public Benefit Corporation (MAPS PBC), and currently serves as Training Manager at Alma Institute.

Her involvement in psychedelics is deeply guided by her advocacy for and commitment to harm-reduction principles; trauma-informed care; healing justice; and building community resilience, reciprocity, and accountability within the psychedelic space. Juliette penned a brilliant paper entitled "Psychedelic Extractivism: Distilling Indigeneity into Exchange Value," which heavily informed the content of these chapters. You can read it in its entirety and explore the topics raised by visiting her website.[1]

Limitations: I am writing primarily for an audience of readers participating in the psychedelic resurgence, which spans many groups and a wide spectrum of lived experience that cannot be generalized. The current momentum around psychedelics is centralized in the United States and parts of Europe. Due to issues we will discuss in these chapters, a majority of this audience consists of people who do not have direct lived experience of Indigeneity and the specific, historical, and ongoing oppression endured by these communities.

I offer my deep gratitude to tribal members and Indigenous medicine keepers and leaders from around the world who have chosen to give of their time and energy to educate and guide the psychedelic field in our efforts toward right relationship, some of whom I have the honor to be deepening personal relationships with.

Throughout the text, I will attempt to be clear about whom I am referring to when I say "we/us." Generally speaking, the use of we/us in these chapters refers to Westerners engaging with psychedelics outside of their own ancestral contexts. This language is not meant to further separate the psychedelic field from Indigenous wisdom traditions, but rather to be explicit about the distinct ways that different people groups are impacted by the growing interest in and globalization of entheogenic substances and sacred practice.

WEAVING PSYCHEDELIC AND DRUG WAR HISTORY

In order for us to ground into a meaningful dialogue about healing, we have to spend time coming to terms with the context in which our lives are set—our collective and individual histories. We have been directly and indirectly shaped by infinite past events that have occurred, and we participate in shaping the events that play out now, writing the history of these times. Learning to value history and context helps us support deeper personal, collective, and intergenerational healing, gain understanding, and prevent harm.

As a parent, I remember many times hearing my small son crying from the other room. I would run in, scoop him up, and instinctively, the first question I would ask is, *"What happened?"* This question is essential to our understanding of what needs healing and how to heal it. The same is true within our society and our movements.

The history of psychedelic research and the current resurgence has been told again and again. Unfortunately, that telling often centers Western researchers and fails to look at the larger contexts in which the events of the "psychedelic renaissance" are couched. By stepping back and taking in a larger scope, we open ourselves up to deeper understanding and broader possibilities for healing.

History is often told by the conquerors. Because of this, the information we have access to is filtered through the lens of colonialism. *Colonialism refers to the domination of one culture, society, or nation over another.* The downstream impacts of colonialism are felt in every aspect of contemporary society; we cannot extricate ourselves from this history.

My understanding of history is incomplete. It is also skewed by my lived experience, and by the access I do and do not have to traditional wisdom keepers who can tell their stories in their own languages and perspectives. This chapter is offered with humility and acknowledgment that history is expansive, multifaceted, and cannot be summed up in words written in English in a book.

FORMS OF HISTORY

There are a few forms of history that are important to spend time with when approaching psychedelics. Entire volumes could be written about them, and this book will only scratch the surface. These forms of history include the following.

COLONIAL HISTORY: This is the broader context we collectively find ourselves in at this moment in human history. We are at a peak expression of a global colonial project that began around 1500 and has shaped nearly every facet of life on this planet. This is a historical fact; we live in a colonized world largely controlled by descendants of those who enacted colonization over several centuries.

The motives for colonization were manifold. Key among them were the impulses to increase wealth, control trade routes, spread Christianity, and become the dominant world power. Beneath these expressed intentions was the willingness to commit racial and cultural genocide, the method by which these capitalist and religious aims were achieved. Because these efforts were so abhorrent, violent, and completely lacking in logic, a mythology had to be created to justify them. What resulted was the creation of a racial hierarchy that placed white colonists as "superior" to the People of the Global Majority (PGM). Thus, racial capitalism came to exist, a system that has been perpetuated around the world for over five hundred years.[2]

The term (and framework) *racial capitalism* was originally established by political science and Black Studies professor Cedric Robinson, who extensively researched the historical forces and conditions that created capitalism.[3] For him, racial capitalism meant that capitalism has been inseparably linked to ideas of race and racism throughout its history. Capitalism built up its wealth from the transatlantic slave trade and colonial exploitation.[4]

He states that "racial regimes are constructed social systems in which race is proposed as a justification for the relations of power." He continues:

> As Western European nations overtook control of various areas, leaders and merchants moved many indigenous peoples from their homelands to solve labor shortages faced by the colonial powers. The African slave trade is the example that comes to mind for most people, but other peoples were also enslaved, e.g., Chinese and Indian. The slave trade was possible because there was a belief that anyone not living in the manner of Western Europeans was inherently backward or lesser than white Europeans. This *dehumanization,* or denial of humanness, was essential to colonial practices as it provided a justification for aggressive and morally questionable practices.[5]

It can be argued that *racial capitalism* is really just another term for *capitalism.* It is a system grounded in the extraction of social and economic value from people of marginalized racial identities. Scholar Jodi Melamed states that capitalism "can only accumulate by producing and moving through relations of severe inequality among human groups," and therefore, for capitalism to survive, it must exploit and prey upon the "unequal differentiation of human value."[6]

Colonial systems are not laws of nature, and as such, we can return to healthier ways of being as we move forward. These systems are best understood as a structure, process, or project, because it reveals the concerted and ongoing human effort of designing, constructing, carrying out, and maintaining the project of colonialism across the globe.

Latin American activist and scholar Manuela Picq writes:

> Colonialism is a structure, not an event. Patrick Wolfe argued that invasion is not an isolated historical event because settlers come to stay and proposed to think of it as a structuring principle. Colonialism is an ongoing process that still defines borders between imagined centers and peripheries, and the doctrine of discovery remains foundational to the international system of states built on stolen Indigenous lands. This violent process is not a left-over from the past, it is a core principle necessary to the survival of the current state system.[7]

At this point, we are embedded within colonial structures that come with specific harms, power dynamics, and narratives attached to them. This is the context in which the "psychedelic renaissance" is unfolding.

LIVING HISTORY: This is the history of the Indigenous communities who steward the medicines that are now gaining popularity among non-Native groups. In addition to their unique generations-old relationships with powerful medicines like peyote, psilocybin, ayahuasca, and iboga—to name a few—there is a deeper medicine tied up with this living history. The medicines are not only the plants, mushrooms, and sacred brews we now venerate. The medicines we desperately need in these times of crisis are the lifeways, knowledge, and traditions that teach humans how to live on this planet in a good way. That is the medicine held intact by Indigenous communities around the world. It is a symptom of colonial thought to reduce the rich history of Indigenous communities to only the aspects that interest oneself. This is why conversations about reciprocity are so often problematic and counterproductive; because when trying to translate reciprocity into accessible practice, they reduce an Indigenous concept of grounded relational exchange to a distant transactional act. This disregards the larger context from which the healing practices emerge.

Around the world, Indigenous communities have and continue to face similar struggles under the forces of the global colonial project. Recognizing these patterns causes us to take a sober look at the undercurrents and belief systems driving this project.

MEDICINE HISTORY: Each medicine we work with, whether it emerged from a plant, a fungus, or a chemical reaction, has a story. What were, in many cases, held as sacraments and integral parts of the human experience for centuries, were then demonized and treated as a threat to colonial control. These practices threatened the assimilating and extinguishing project of colonialism as these medicines were originally deeply rooted in cultural tradition and community relationships. Furthermore, the era of prohibition and criminalization is tied up with the efforts to eradicate the culture, spirituality, and autonomy of conquered peoples.

That era is also tied up in the broader efforts to suppress consciousness. The ability of an oppressive capitalist system to maintain itself begins to crumble when the populace wakes up to the realities of their own participation in what is making them sick. This is part of the power of expanded states of consciousness—they can wake us up to memories, realities, and possibilities beyond the structures we currently find ourselves in. This is dangerous in the best way. It is also why we have to be careful and highly intentional with how we approach policy change. Incremental change that is framed in benefits rather than deconstruction is less likely to be met with opposition from existing power structures. This is steady, gradual work.

GENERATIONAL HISTORY: As discussed in chapter 1, about Inner-Work, the generational wounds we carry and the impacts of systems we are embedded within are present within people of all backgrounds. A great part of the healing path is getting into relationship with the roots of our stories, which extend far back beyond our parents and grandparents. Our generational history is the story of lineage. For many of us, it is the story of many lineages converging, and all of the beautiful and horrific events that were wrapped up in that unfolding that ultimately led to you. It is also a contemplation of who and which lineages were *not allowed to continue* due to colonial violence, which lineages have been erased, and which lineages are here today because they resisted and survived against a system that intended to push them into extinction.

Generational history is more than a tale of historical trauma and struggle. It is an epic tale of land, wars, culture, spirituality, ceremony, tradition, magic, language, plants, animals, and a sense of place. It is the story of the medicine carriers who held knowledge of the foods and herbs and waters where the ancestors found a home. It is the stories they told around the fires and the contented silence of the ordinary in-between moments.

These are truths we can never know for certain, but can feel in our bones because our cells remember that these lives were lived. Our generational history is a reminder that there is life beyond violent struggles for power. Because our ancestors experienced it and they are our through line to return. If we get quiet enough, if we go far enough back, we can find it. We can continue in the footsteps of the lives that we hoped and expected to live before humans set out to conquer one another.

BIOGRAPHICAL HISTORY: This brings us to today. Small, marvelous you, with all the winding paths that converged and resulted in your life. Your biographical history is your story. It is the context in which your life has unfolded and the factors that shaped it. It is the joys and heartaches, traumatic experiences, and profound wonders. Your history is likely a driving factor in your choice to work with psychedelic and plant medicines. It is often where we begin a conversation with them. It is the immediate experience. Your story is often the starting point in journey work and the first site of what you'll unpack when you begin to heal.

History in the Medicine Space

There is an inherent tension for those of us in the psychedelic field who live in the United States. This is a nation materially and ideologically built upon Indigenous genocide and the enslavement of African people. This is a nation that set in motion what has become a global drug war, originally to assert control over communities of color and those opposed to the Vietnam War. This country is also situated at the center of the resurgence of altered states and the most likely beneficiary of psychedelic commercialization. Because of this entanglement, we can't have a conversation about history and healing with integrity without discussing these hard truths.

In a talk for Psychedelic Seminars in 2020, Camille Barton said that:

> Colonialism is a historical event, but it lives on in our actions, our bodies, and the ways that Westerners often feel entitled to take from other communities without reciprocity. This desperately needs to shift if we are going to create a more equitable world and shape drug policy to benefit people who have been harmed by the legacies of colonization and disproportionately impacted by the war on drugs and the incarceration and the destruction of families this has created.[8]

THE DRUG WAR

An in-depth look at the history of the drug war is beyond the scope of this book; however, there are numerous resources available to understand its events, nuances, and the ways they impact us today. These include the Drug Policy Alliance and books such as *The New Jim Crow* by Michelle Alexander, *Chasing the Scream* by Johann Hari, and *Drug Use for Grown-Ups* by Dr. Carl Hart.

At a Glance

Richard Nixon famously declared drugs "public enemy number one" in 1971. This catalyzed a fifty-year drug war that targeted Black, Indigenous, Latino, poor, and other marginalized communities—despite their sharing similar rates of use with white communities. It resulted in the United States having the largest prison population in the world, and a thriving global black market worth half a trillion dollars.[9] The drug war has been a driving factor in increased police brutality and has been utilized as a pipeline to force community members into the prison and legal system, which has lifelong and intergenerational consequences.

According to the Drug Policy Alliance:

- Nearly 80% of people in federal prison and almost 60% of people in state prison for drug offenses are Black or Latino.

- Research shows that prosecutors are twice as likely to pursue a mandatory minimum sentence for Black people as for white people charged with the same offense. Among people who received a mandatory minimum sentence in 2011, 38% were Latino and 31% were Black.

- Black people and Native Americans are more likely to be killed by law enforcement than other racial or ethnic groups. They are often stereotyped as being violent or addicted to alcohol and other drugs. Experts believe that stigma and racism might play a major role in police-community interactions.

Punishment for a drug law violation is not only meted out by the criminal legal system, but is also perpetuated by policies denying child custody, voting rights, employment, business loans, licensing, student aid, public housing, and other public assistance to people with criminal convictions.

These exclusions create a permanent second-class status for millions of Americans. Like drug war enforcement itself, they fall disproportionately on people of color.[10]

A War on Us

The United States drug war, which began as early as 1890, took shape in the 1930s with Harry Anslinger's Bureau of Narcotics, and continued to proliferate under Richard Nixon, Ronald Reagan, and Bill Clinton. Over time, the US government crafted a strategic narrative that demonized nonwhite communities and bolstered support for the policies that became the cornerstones of the drug war. These tactics included criminalizing substances such as opium, cannabis, crack cocaine, and many Indigenous medicines due to their connections to communities of color. In the United States, designing extremely disproportionate drug possession punishments between coca's derivatives, powder and crack cocaine (100 grams of powdered cocaine held the same legal punishment as 1 gram of crack cocaine), led to the arrests and incarceration of Black people en masse, while white users of powdered cocaine were punished less.

In regard to Indigenous Medicine, the Religious Crimes Act of 1883 banned Native dances, ceremonies, and medicine practices. The code gave Indian agents authority to use force, imprisonment, and the withholding of rations to stop any cultural practices they deemed immoral or subversive to federal government-mandated assimilation policies. The return of these basic civil liberties was not enacted until 1978, almost a hundred years later, with the American Indian Religious Freedom Act. Peyote use was not legally protected for the Native American Church until the act was amended in 1994.

PSYCHEDELIC EXCEPTIONALISM

Within the psychedelic field, there is a risk of participating in what is known as psychedelic exceptionalism. The practice of categorizing substances as good and bad is prevalent within the psychedelic world, and represents a double standard that condemns some substances, and the people who consume them, while celebrating others. Not only is this an arbitrary form of evaluation that is totally subjective and based on personal and collective bias; it also causes us to pour a great deal of energy and resources into ending the criminalization of psychedelic substances (or those to which we assign the label of psychedelic), which have relatively low rates of arrest, while validating and upholding the criminalization of the substances actually driving mass incarceration (cocaine, heroin, cannabis, and amphetamines).

For example, MDMA, embraced by the FDA as a breakthrough therapy and at the heart of the mainstreaming of psychedelics, *is an amphetamine.* This further illustrates that we cannot easily classify drugs as medicine versus problematic; there are many contextual factors impacting whether a drug has beneficial, neutral, or harmful effects on someone, and none of those factors have any bearing on whether people who use drugs should be criminalized and locked in cages.

Even though I was exposed to the sale and functional use of prohibited substances throughout my youth, it took me years to unpack my own conditioning around drugs. It's important to be patient with ourselves and those around us during the unlearning process; many of us were indoctrinated during the peak of the drug war, from Nancy Reagan's "Just Say No" efforts and the "This is your brain on drugs" campaigns of the 1980s, to the fear-fueled DARE classes I sat through in the 1990s. There are a lot of mistruths to unlearn. When we return to our logic and our humanity, we can access many more effective, humane, and systemic solutions to address problematic drug use in our society.

Because of the mainstream spotlight on the movement to legalize psychedelics, those of us in positions of influence need to leverage every opportunity to frame this work within the larger context of dismantling the unjust drug war. Part of our cultural healing will hinge on us all working together to unravel the harms of the drug war on all fronts: in policy, society, and our communities and families.

COLONIALISM IN PSYCHEDELIC PLANT MEDICINES
The Stories We Tell

The telling of history is not unbiased. Human engagement with psychedelic plants goes back many thousands, if not millions, of years. It is also inseparable from a recent historical context shaped by colonial domination and imperialism. It should come as no surprise then that the "origin stories" of psilocybin mushrooms, peyote, and ayahuasca are fraught with a classic colonial tale: one of contact, "discovery," appropriation, assimilation, exploitation, and extraction. Then came the erasure of that history. Through this erasure, Indigenous peoples and their cultures were cast as something exotic and "ancient," existing only in the past. In recent decades, psychedelics were so far removed from their Indigenous origins and instead associated only with Western male researchers and white hippie counterculture that many communities of color, living through the violence of the drug war, rejected these substances and viewed them as dangerous.

When colonial settlers first encountered Indigenous peoples practicing their traditional ceremonies, these practices were demonized and pushed into the shadows by settlers. For example, the use of peyote was banned for the Aztec people by Spanish colonists in 1620. It represented a threat to the colonial project of civilizing and purifying Indigenous bodies and forced conversions to Christianity. Spanish colonists associated psilocybin mushroom use with devil worship, and in the first written accounts of ayahuasca use, Jesuit missionaries wrote that ayahuasca "serves for mystification and bewitchment . . . for superstitious practices and witchcraft."[11]

A lot has changed since then; white communities now venerate the medicines that many of their ancestors demonized. In order to heal and move forward, we must reckon with our own contradictions. Otherwise, this is how colonialism is perpetuated: by refusing to acknowledge the ways we benefit from the erasure, extraction, exploitation, and appropriation of Indigenous peoples and their customs. We have an opportunity to walk a new path so that the stories told of these times are accounts of healing, repair, and restoration.

Below is a brief look at some of the prominent entheogens and substances gaining popularity amid the "psychedelic renaissance." The following list is by no means exhaustive. It's important to remember that many entheogens are found throughout multiple continents and their practices vary between lineages. Additionally, much history has been lost and erased through the process of colonization. While I hope the information below is helpful, it lacks the rich cultural history that is held within Indigenous communities about their medicines and is only theirs to share.

PSILOCYBIN

Psilocybin mushrooms have confirmed Indigenous roots in Central America, most notably the Mazatec people of Oaxaca, Mexico, as well as the Mixtec, Nashua, and Zapotec peoples. Ancient Greeks used a combination of psychedelic mushrooms and ergot fungus in their ceremonial brews. Evidence of ceremonial mushroom use has also been found in Africa, with Algerian cave paintings dating back 9,000 years and *Psilocybe* mushrooms found in Central Africa and South Sudan.

Contemporary Mazatec people have spoken of the "Hippie Invasion" of the 1960s and the way the commodification of sacred mushrooms reshaped their communities:

> The arrival of foreigners took place in a complex historical context
> because, alongside the arrival of the counterculture movement in the

1960s, increasing numbers of roads and highways were being built in the Sierra Mazateca at the time. These opened a remote, mountainous region evermore to capitalist logic and government initiatives, further facilitating the arrival of *güeros,* as tourists are called. Over the years, a special kind of tourism began to develop, catering to those who sought to have contact with the "little ones" and the *Chjon Chjine* or *Chjota Chjine,* inspired by the magazine story about María Sabina. She became a key figure for outsiders, but was ostracized and reproached by her community for revealing the secret of the mushrooms.[12]

We will spend more time with María Sabina's story in the coming chapter.

HUACHUMA

Known as the grandfather of entheogens, Huachuma (which came to be known as San Pedro after the Spanish Invasion) is a cactus native to Peru and Bolivia, with use tracing back 4,000 years. This medicinal plant is associated with the Chavín culture of the Andes, which laid the foundations for the Inca civilization. Stone temple slabs dating back to 1,300 BCE show a figure holding a Huachuma cactus, pointing to its cultural significance.

Huachuma contains mescaline, and while it is legal in the United States to grow the cactus for ornamental purposes, consuming mescaline is illegal. Because it grows so much faster than peyote and is more widely available, conservation and Indigenous rights advocates urge those who feel called toward a relationship with mescaline to choose to work with huachuma rather than peyote. In this way we can preserve peyote in solidarity with the Native American communities for whom it is a sacrament.

RAPÉ

Tobacco is one of the oldest and most important ceremonial medicines in the Americas, and among the more stigmatized plant medicines due to humans' complicated relationship with it. It is impossible to separate Indigenous history in the Americas from the ceremonial use of tobacco, known as *mapacho*. Rapé (pronounced "ha-peh," also called hapé or rapéh) is a form of sacred Amazonian snuff tobacco. It is made by combining dried tobacco leaves *(Nicotiana rustica)* with sacred tree ash and other botanicals and grinding it into a dust-fine powder. Blends are distinct from tribe to tribe and the process of making rapé can take several weeks. It is known for its grounding and stimulating qualities.

Tobacco is not prohibited in most of the world the way other entheogens are. However, this open legal market has created other concerns. In recent years, an explosion in global interest in rapé has resulted in many white-owned "shamanic supply" businesses popping up online, selling rapé and other Amazonian medicines on web stores and Instagram. It is wise to dig deeper when companies claim they are in partnership with local tribes or have a "trusted source." Keep in mind that "a portion of proceeds returned to the tribes" and "mutually beneficial relationship" are undefined and potentially exploitative claims and fair trade practices aren't always readily enforced.

IBOGAINE

Ibogaine is a powerful medicine that comes from the root bark of the iboga shrub, native to Gabon in central West Africa. It has been used for centuries by people of the Bwiti tradition as a rite of passage and initiation. The preservation and expansion of the Bwiti practice and iboga medicine have a complex history involving French occupation, displacement, intertribal violence, religious suppression, and political marginalization.[13]

Medicalization of ibogaine began in the late 1930s with decades of intermittent yet promising research into its potential to treat substance use disorders, particularly opiate addiction. Its legal status remains complicated and restricted in many countries.

Global enthusiasm about iboga's healing potential has created problems not unlike those faced by Indigenous Americans with peyote, such as difficulty sourcing medicine for their traditional use and ongoing political struggle to protect their practices.

Wild iboga is currently endangered in Gabon due to poaching, climate change, illegal export to satisfy international demand, urbanization, and habitat degradation. As an alternative, iboga can be grown sustainably in greenhouses and farms, and advocates also point to the option of using semi-synthetic ibogaine from the *Voacanga africana* tree instead.

DMT

DMT has been called "the spirit molecule." This powerful, naturally occurring entheogen is concentrated in modern ayahuasca brew, thanks to the presence of chacruna leaves. It is also produced endogenously by a variety of plants, fungi, and animals—including toads, salamanders, rats, shrubs, seeds, and amanita mushrooms. Humans even produce it at birth and death, and it has been found in the urine of people experiencing schizophrenia and other psychoses. DMT is structurally similar to LSD.

Due to conservation concerns, many in the psychedelic field advocate for the use of synthetically derived DMT to avoid contributing to habitat loss and extinction as interest in this medicine grows.

LSD

While tiny squares of paper blotted with synthesized LSD and printed with cartoon characters may seem the farthest thing from nature, it was first discovered by Swiss chemist Albert Hoffman working with ergot, a fungus that grows on rye.

OTHER LAB-MADE TEACHERS

Synthesized compounds such as MDMA, ketamine, 2C-B, and others need not be excluded from the list of substances deserving of our gratitude. When we partake with intentionality, the journeys give generously back to us. Sacred reciprocity can be viewed as an essential element of psychedelic experience, regardless of the catalyzing substance. It is beneficial to relate to everything that sustains and heals us from the paradigm of relationship rather than utility.

Medicines of the Resistance

In *Our History Is the Future: Standing Rock Versus the Dakota Access Pipeline, and the Long Tradition of Indigenous Resistance,* prominent Indigenous activist Nick Estes (of the Lower Brule Sioux Tribe) writes that "Indigenous resistance draws from a long history, projecting itself backward and forward in time. While traditional historians merely interpret the past, radical Indigenous historians and Indigenous knowledge-keepers aim to change the colonial present, and to imagine a decolonial future by reconnecting to Indigenous places and histories. For this to occur, those suppressed practices must make a crack in history."[14]

Traditional medicines such as peyote and ayahuasca played a key role in the collective healing, spiritual survival, and political resistance of the Indigenous peoples who stewarded them during periods of colonization and forced assimilation.

PEYOTE

Peyote is a sacred cactus native to what is now known as the American Southwest, Mexico, and Peru. With a human–plant relationship dating back 10,000 years, this ceremonial cactus has been used in rites of passage and annual pilgrimages by Native American and Mexican Indigenous groups for millennia. It is inseparable from cultural heritage for many tribes, including the Wixárika, Rarámuri, Yaqui, and Cora peoples.

Peyote contains mescaline, a psychoactive substance also found in Huachuma (San Pedro cactus). Outlawed by the Spanish Inquisition in 1620, peyote was the first substance ever criminalized in the Americas. For the last century, Indigenous groups in North America have fought convoluted government policies, environmental degradation, private land ownership, poaching, mining, and urbanization in their efforts to preserve their spiritual practice.

Boarding schools in North America were utilized as sites of removal of Native children, dispossession, death, murder, and cultural and physical genocide. Peyote acted as a force of healing, cultural sovereignty, bonding, and resistance. Peyote use spread through Mexican and American Indigenous communities in the second half of the nineteenth century within colonial boarding schools. Peyote was shared within secret networks, acting as an escape from white impositions, and utilized as a medicine and a sacrament.[15]

The Kiowa tribe used peyote to treat tuberculosis, saving the lives of many students returning from boarding schools. James Mooney documented that these students were the most outspoken defenders of the peyote ceremony, having experienced medicinal relief and healing.[16]

The development of the peyote religious movement can be seen as an Indigenous spiritual resistance movement to the United States' ethnocide, or the deliberate destruction of culture, where "the ability and strength to handle the trauma of cultural and social disintegration wrought by the reservation system and policies of forced acculturation were necessary for the survival of individuals, families, and communities of Native peoples."[17]

The peyote tradition's focus on community and cultural preservation offered an opportunity for individual and collective healing that was adept at meeting the needs of reservation communities. Peyote then spread across reservations in the US, emerging as a healing practice and a critical cultural resource that played a large role in the expansion of the Native American Church (NAC), eventually growing to be the largest intertribal Indigenous religion in the United States.

Peyote supported spiritual and cultural resistance to ethnocide. Peyote can thus be understood as a spiritual and medicinal plant ally that aided Indigenous peoples' survival and resistance during times of extreme colonial violence and cultural suppression, and continues to play a critical role in the resurgence of Indigenous ways of life across Turtle Island, known as North America.

Peyote: Current Challenges

This precious medicine is currently under threat. Peyote is an endangered species in its US habitat and multiple converging factors are contributing to a drastic decline in supply. This correlates to a sharp increase in price and limits the access and quality of peyote buttons that are available to members of the Native American Church today. "Peyote is part of a whole; it is not merely a plant," remarks Wixárika lawyer Santos Rentería. "It is a being that is part of an ecological and cultural landscape dating back millennia. All elements affecting the individual peyote are also transforming the landscape as a whole. In the end, both the landscape and the individual plant are under threat, and their conservation must attend to this symbiotic factor."[18] The colonial history of the land is intertwined with the spread of the peyote tradition: the creation of the US–Mexico border, the conversion of the land to private property, the removal of Native Americans to reservations, and the expansion of the United States all facilitated conditions that have made peyote an integral yet scarce resource for the NAC way of life.

Peyote's habitat range in the United States is restricted to a narrow strip of land along the US–Mexico border in Southwestern Texas that is only between 5,180 and 6,475 square kilometers. In the only place where peyote grows in the United States—South Texas's Zapata, Webb, and Starr counties—construction of Trump's border wall further devastated the ecosystem. The implications of colonial domination on peyote and the ecosystem it is embedded within continue to affect its growth, cultivation, distribution, and cultural use.

The Indigenous Peyote Conservation Initiative (IPCI) is an Indigenous-led collaborative effort to preserve peyote and ensure the survival of this sacred practice for generations to come. We will discuss this more in the following chapter, 12, about Reciprocity.

AYAHUASCA

Ayahuasca spread throughout Amazonian communities during the boom of the rubber tapping industries, historically noted as an era of intense destruction, tragedy, and exploitation for the Amazon forest peoples. During this time, Indigenous groups were enslaved and dislocated, and experienced mass death due to disease.[19]

Thousands of Amazon forest people died in a very short time as a result of the murder, abuse, and disease brought on by the rubber trade, and in many circumstances, traditional healing preparations such as ayahuasca and other medicinal plants were the only resources available to these communities for healing.

In his influential tome *Shamanism, Colonialism, and the Wild Man: A Study in Terror and Healing,* Michael Taussig recognizes the rise of ayahuasca shamanism during a time when Indigenous communities were stripped of their traditions and "transformed into labor for the global industry" as an extension of the "disorderly brutality of colonialism and capitalist expansion."[20] He was especially interested in how notions of the "primitive" and images of the "wild Indian" were projected onto Indigenous groups and Indigenous healing practices by Western colonists and capitalists during this time of encounter.

Ayahuasca: Current Challenges

In recent decades, ayahuasca tourism in the Amazon has become a surging market, which has presented economic benefits and cultural challenges for Amazon forest communities. Maestro (medicine person/healer) Pedro Tangoa López claims that ayahuasca tourism and commercialization are distorting the cultural originality and traditions of the medicine, contributing to a "huge cultural devastation." Maestra Vicky Corisepa laments, "Our culture has been disappearing, due to all the transnational invasions green-lit by the government. It is disrespecting the Native people."[21] Maestro López also voices concerns about overharvesting of ayahuasca, causing scarcity and fears of deforestation in local areas: "If we don't do anything, I think that in ten to fifteen years we're going to be talking as we did with the disappearance of mahogany in the Amazon."[22] The declining supply of local ayahuasca has caused prices of the *Banisteriopsis caapi* vine to more than triple between 2012 to 2017 with younger and thinner vines used more than ever to keep up with tourist demand.[23]

Patenting Ayahuasca

Ayahuasca itself was patented in 1986 by an American citizen named Loren Miller, director of the International Plant Medicine company based in California. He applied for the patent in 1984, ten years after being given a sample of the *B. caapi* vine by an Indigenous leader in Ecuador.[24] In response to plant patent 5,751, the Coordinator of the Indigenous Organizations of the Amazon River Basin (COICA), representing over four hundred Indigenous communities across that region, criticized the plunder and disrespect of the sacred symbol and, alongside the Center for International Environmental Law (CIEL), requested a reexamination of the patent.[25]

The patent reexamination highlighted requirements that a plant must be new and distinct in order to be considered patentable as well as arguing for a case of biopiracy and invoking a moral utility doctrine to prevent the theft of Indigenous community-held knowledge. The patent was rejected in 1999, citing lack of novelty yet rejecting the claims of biopiracy and moral utility. Loren Miller appealed, and the US Patent and Trademark Office sided with Miller's appeal, reinstating plant patent 5,751 in 2001, lasting for the remaining two years of its term.[26]

In the 2019 Pronouncement of the Shipibo-Konibo-Xetebo Nation on the Globalization of Ayahuasca, the Shipibo-Konibo-Xetebo Association of Onanyabo/Ancestral Healers cited "rampant abuse of our sacred plants and of the ancestral knowledge of Amazonian Peoples," stating that they are "tired of seeing our knowledge and ancestral practices appropriated by a cannibalistic Western system."[27]

RECKONING WITH HISTORY

These are the contexts we must know and reckon with as enthusiasm for yagé or ayahuasca grows. The echoes of María Sabina's story in Huautla de Jiménez are undeniable—a tangle of sincere interest and extractive intentions descended upon the local communities in search of an "exotic" medicine to heal the wounds of Westerners, and forever changed the community. It is impossible for outsiders to enter a place or culture and consume it without impacting the lived realities of those who live there. Our actions hold unintended consequences. Is it possible to make peace with this? How do we reconcile with the psychedelic tourism phenomenon that provides economic support to peoples of the Amazon but simultaneously results in extraction of their medicine, competition between medicine people and profiteers, and cultural degradation? What does a truth and reconciliation process look like with these communities? These are questions we need to grapple with as a field and center in our discourses.

At the very least, we can begin by listening deeply to the concerns, requests, and direction of Indigenous leaders. We can prioritize Indigenous access to their own medicines. *We can resist the continued forces of colonialism that position traditional medicine-keepers as tokens to lend legitimacy to white-owned organizations and retreat centers.* We can contribute to Indigenous-led conservation efforts. We can form sincere and lasting partnerships directly with Indigenous-led projects to advance their priorities, needs, goals, and dreams. We can move slowly, listen, build relationships, and take the months and years required to comprehend the complex sociopolitical dynamics impacting the globalization of sacred medicines.

As of this writing, Alma Institute and Fungi Foundation have been partnering in one such closely held relationship. We are working to support a project led by the Mazatec scholar and historian, Inti García Flores, the steward of María Sabina's archives and personal effects. He and his community are asking the psychedelic field to support their efforts to create a Mazatec cultural center in Huautla de Jiménez that will preserve these precious historical and cultural artifacts.

This center will provide a central hub for all generations to rediscover and celebrate their heritage, and cultivate medicinal gardens where the community can reestablish relationships with their ancestral plants. This is just one example of the Indigenous-led efforts the global psychedelic community can support as we seek to understand and protect the past and present histories of these life-changing medicines. You can learn more and support the Historias y Memorias Mazatecas project through the Fungi Foundation.[28]

INDIGENOUS RESISTANCE

The late 1960s in the United States weren't only defined by the launch of the militarized drug war. The Native American movement for resurgence, sovereignty, and self-determination also gained momentum alongside the civil rights movement and antiwar effort. Although Indigenous nations across the Americas have always resisted settler colonialism, this period was a crucial time for the growth and public expression of Indigenous resistance and movement building. Many of these resistance efforts centered on accessing basic needs like food, housing, healthcare, and legal protections, as well as fighting ongoing discrimination, police brutality, unemployment, and criminalization of Native spiritual practices. They sought to build power and collaboration among Native groups and bring into public consciousness the failures of the federal government to honor the hundreds of treaties that had been made.

From this foundation, the American Indian Movement (AIM) was birthed by tribal activists and rapidly gained hundreds of members. The subsequent Indigenous (re)occupations of Alcatraz Island (1969–1971), Mount Rushmore (1971), and Wounded Knee (1973) raised global awareness of the ongoing injustices faced by the Indigenous peoples of Turtle Island at the hands of the US federal government. The American Indian Movement made its way across the United States with the Trail of Broken Treaties demonstration in 1972, where a caravan of Indian activists traveled from California to Washington DC, crossing through many reservations and urban Indian communities to draw national attention to the grievances of Native Americans.

The Trail of Broken Treaties further engaged Native communities in the struggle for liberation with the AIM 20-Point Position paper[29] emerging out of this cross-country caravan, focusing on systemic changes that would impact Native communities. Many of these points concentrate on the restoration of treaties, asserting Indigenous sovereignties, changing the governance of reservations, and abolishing the Bureau of Indian Affairs (BIA). They also contributed to a cultural shift in which Indigenous peoples regained pride in their heritage and were emboldened in their resistance to forced assimilation and cultural erasure.

Efforts toward justice and repair have ebbed and flowed in visibility throughout recent decades, but have never been extinguished. Today many examples of contemporary Indigenous resistance are a continuous demonstration of the strength, resilience, and dignity of Indigenous peoples.

Indigenous Resistance Today

Indigenous peoples still stand in defense of their lands, relationships and life-ways: "as they have always done."

—MANUELA PICQ[30]

MMIWG2S+

The Missing and Murdered Indigenous Women, Girls, and Two-Spirit People campaign (MMIWG2S+) is a movement that seeks to address and end the ongoing disparate acts of violence and genocide experienced by Indigenous women, girls, transgender, gender-diverse, and two-spirit people in Canada. These people in the United States and Canada experience alarmingly higher rates of violence and homicide compared to non-Native counterparts.[31] The Native Women's Association of Canada (NWAC) 2019 report made clear connections between violence and erosion of sovereignty, colonial child welfare policies, and poverty resulting from exploitation of resources and bodies.

Colonial systems have eroded protections for the safety of Native women by limiting tribes' jurisdiction over crimes committed by non-Indians, meaning accountability and justice are controlled by the colonizer state. NWAC's "Reclaiming Power and Place" report[32] highlights a revitalization framework that works toward healing individuals and communities. The new framework includes centering relationships, Indigenous recognitions of power and place, emphasizing accountability, and understanding colonization as gendered oppression. It also affirms Indigenous women's right to culture, health, security, and justice, and looks to state accountability for the lack of justice for these cases.

THE RED NATION

The Red Nation is a movement born out of racial and police violence against Indigenous community members. It formed in New Mexico in 2014 to address the "marginalization and invisibility of Native struggles within mainstream social justice organizing, and to foreground the targeted destruction and violence towards Native life and land." The Red Nation Manifesto established a ten-point program demanding an end to violence against Native peoples and nonhuman relatives, focused on four areas of struggle: Indigeneity, Liberation, Resistance, and Coalition.

The Red Nation asserts that Native people "must first be afforded dignified lives as Native peoples who are free to perform our purpose as stewards of life if we are to protect and respect our nonhuman relatives—the land, the water, the plants, and the animals. We experience the destruction and violation of our non-human relatives wrought by militarization, toxic dumping and contamination, and resource extraction as violent."[33] In many ways, Indigenous struggles for liberation, revitalization, and resurgence are fundamentally tied to the protection of and responsibility to life itself—life of community, life of other-than-human kin, and life of land.

INDIGENOUS LAND, WATER, AND AIR DEFENDERS

There is an established history of Indigenous-led defense of sacred lands against environmental harms. In 1981, the Fort McDowell Yavapai Nation of Arizona successfully won a struggle against the construction of the Orme Dam, a federal dam project that threatened to flood more than half of the Fort McDowell Yavapai Reservation's ancestral land and a majority of their farmland. An Indigenous-led coalition formed in 2004 to defend the San Francisco Peaks, land that is sacred and has significant cultural meaning for many regions' Indigenous tribes, from development by the Arizona Snowbowl ski resort. The Protect the Peaks coalition protested the "clearcutting of approximately 30,000 trees, that is home to threatened species, making new runs and lifts, more parking lots, and building a 14.8-mile buried pipeline to transport up to 180 million gallons (per season) of wastewater to make artificial snow on 205 acres."[34]

Indigenous groups in 2011 campaigned against the Keystone XL Pipeline project, a proposed 1,700-mile oil pipeline that would have carried oil from Canada all the way to the Gulf of Mexico. The proposed site of the pipeline crossed waterways, sacred sites, and burial grounds of the Fort Belknap Indian Reservation. In 2016, the Standing Rock Sioux protested against the Dakota Access Pipeline (DAPL), a 1,100-mile pipeline connecting to another pipeline that transports 450,000 barrels of oil per day to the Gulf of Mexico. The pipeline was rerouted from an original proposed path running near Bismarck, North Dakota, to instead run beneath Mni Sose (Missouri River) and through Oceti Sakowin treaty lands and the Standing Rock Sioux Reservation. The pipeline threatened to destroy sacred homeland, with potential oil leaks at risk of poisoning not only the tribe's only water supply, but also the risk of polluting the Ogallala Aquifer (one of the largest aquifers in the world) and the Missouri River. The DAPL continues to run, putting the Standing Rock Sioux's resources and livelihood at risk. Other pipeline projects challenged by Indigenous groups include the Line 5 pipeline in Michigan and the Enbridge Line 3 pipeline in Minnesota.

The Unist'ot'en Camp is an Indigenous reoccupation camp and healing center on unceded Wet'suwet'en land. There, defending the land, water, and air goes hand in hand with healing, with a central value being: "Heal the people. Heal the land." For years, Unist'ot'en Camp has been successfully resisting tar sands and fracking gas pipelines proposed by Chevron, Enbridge, and TransCanada through asserting their ancestral stewardship and reciprocal obligations to care for their land and reestablishing traditional protocols for entry— such as checkpoints where they turn away employees of surveyors and those involved in pipeline construction. The camp has turned into a "whole community in resistance," where volunteers have built a healing and cultural center, created a permaculture garden, and host annual action camps. Freda Hudson speaks about the healing center and the responsibility of reciprocity with the land as caretakers and stewards:

> We decided to build this healing centre to bring our own people out here and bring healing to them, spiritually, mentally, physically and use this space to make our people strong. Like the residential schools were used to take the Indian out of the child we want to use this facility to put the Indian back in our children, meaning our culture. If our people have our culture they'll be strong, and they'll be able to stand on their own two feet. And we'll have a strong Nation to learn to take care of ourselves and take care of our resources and take care of the land. And if we take care of the land then the land will take care of us.[35]

The relationship between the land and its people cannot be overstated. When the land experiences harm, so does the community; when the people are displaced, the land suffers. The two are inseparable. This is why we see examples of the same spirited resistance from Indigenous peoples all around the world. To defend the earth is to defend life itself.

HAWAII

Beginning in 2014, Kānaka Maoli kiaʻi (protectors) have resisted the development of the Thirty Meter Telescope (TMT) at the summit of Mauna Kea, the tallest mountain in the world from base to peak. In Kānaka Maoli cosmology, the mountain itself is Wakea, the sky father who played a critical role in the birth/origin story of the Hawaiian Islands. The summit of Mauna Kea is known as the *wao akua* (realm of the gods), home to various deities, as well as sacred burial sites on the mountain. Native Hawaiians share a sacred and ancestral kinship to Mauna Kea and feel a sense of *kuleana* (responsibility) to *mālama* (care for) and protect Mauna Kea from degradation and further development by the settler colonial state.[36] Natural, cultural, and sacred Indigenous Hawaiian resources have been desecrated, lost, and destroyed from previous development and scientific use of the mountain. Since 2014, Indigenous-led Mauna Kea camps have formed and direct action has been employed to stop the construction of the TMT. Kānaka Maoli kia'i are prepared to converge if construction begins again.

THE AMAZON

Indigenous land defenders in the Amazon face violence for their resistance to desecration, degradation, and extraction of their land. In 2018, Olivia Arévalo Lomas—a known ayahuasca *maestra* (medicine woman/healer) and leader of the Shipibo-Konibo Indigenous Amazonian community in Peru—was shot in the chest and killed. The main suspect was her client, a Canadian man. Coordinator of the department of Indigenous communities, Juan Carlos Ruíz Molleda, commented that Maestra Lomas's death constituted "an aggression against the entire Shipibo community," as she "was the living memory of her people."[37] The murder of Maestra Lomas was set within a broader context of conflict between the Shipibo community and extractive corporations encroaching on their ancestral homeland to deforest the Amazon and cultivate palm oil.

The advances of these corporations impact the ability of Amazon forest peoples to subsist on the land as they traditionally have since time immemorial. The degradation of the Peruvian Amazon contaminates waterways and devastates the land, ecosystem, and biodiversity of the Amazon rainforest. "Extractive violence against the land and violence against Indigenous women go hand and hand. We believe that healing women is also healing the earth," proclaims Nina Gualinga of Amazon Watch.[38] Amazon Watch reports increased threats against Indigenous women forest defenders as they stand up to extractive industry and government entities, an increase in gender-based violence, and a lack of public health support for Indigenous peoples during the COVID pandemic.

On International Women's Day 2022, Indigenous women from the Ecuadorian Amazon convened for a march to honor women and land defense threatened by oil and mining corporations, followed by a summit at the Confederation of Indigenous Nationalities of the Ecuadorian Amazon (CONFENIAE) headquarters where they released their Manifesto of Women of the Amazon Indigenous Peoples.

In the manifesto, the women insist that "the full and effective participation and decision-making by women in public life, as well as the elimination of violence, to achieve gender equality and the empowerment of all women and girls is key to action in the Amazon," and denounce

> the state and private violence implemented in the north-central Amazon region, due to the presence of illegal and large-scale mining that directly affects the sovereignty of our territories. We demand our rights to prior consultation and informed consent (FPIC), and the right to self-determination

to be respected, before disposing of our home and desecrating our Mother Earth, because attacking the Amazon is attacking life.[39]

Indigenous women land defenders bring multifaceted solutions to resisting gendered and ecological violence that are intrinsically tied together by colonialism.

LAND BACK

The Land Back movement "[a]dvocates for a transfer of decision-making power over land to Indigenous communities. The movement does not ask current residents to vacate their homes, but maintains that Indigenous governance is possible, sustainable, and preferred for public lands." Land Back, or land restitution, involves relinquishing control and stewardship of land, water, and natural resources, thereby redistributing power and wealth to Indigenous communities. The Land Back movement is "ultimately a manner of securing an Indigenous futurity that includes self-determination, environmental sustainability, and economic justice."[40] The NDN Collective, an Indigenous rights group, describes Land Back as a political framework that represents the reclamation of everything stolen from original peoples, including land, language, ceremony, food, education, housing, healthcare, governance, medicines, and kinship.[41]

Some examples of land returned to Indigenous communities have emerged out of California in recent years. In the California High Sierras, 2,325 acres of ancestral land were transferred back to the Maidu people. The Esselen tribe of Big Sur, California regained 1,200 undeveloped acres of their ancestral homeland in 2020. In September of 2022, the City of Oakland and the Sogorea Te' Land Trust announced a plan to return five acres of land owned by the city, known as Sequoia Point, to Ohlone stewardship. The NDN Collective is focusing their LANDBACK campaign on the closure of Mount Rushmore and repatriation of the Black Hills land in South Dakota.

There are also examples of redistributing resources through a voluntary land tax. The Shuumi Land Tax is a voluntary contribution to support work of the Sogorea Te' Land Trust from settlers living in unceded Lisjan (Ohlone) territory (California's East Bay). *Shuumi* means "gift" in the Ohlone language. The Shuumi Land Tax supports the rematriation of Indigenous land to the Lisjan people, establishing gardens, community and cultural centers, ceremonial spaces, and a cemetery to bury stolen Ohlone ancestral remains—as of this writing, thousands of Ohlone ancestral bones are in the basements of anthropology departments at University of California (UC) Berkeley and San Francisco State University. There is also an Institutional Shuumi Land Tax, and opportunities to volunteer and get engaged with the local Indigenous community. Other existing voluntary land tax programs include Real Rent Duwamish in Seattle, and Wiyot Honor Tax in Northern California. While land tax/rent payments are not an alternative to land restitution, these voluntary contributions redistribute wealth and resources back to Indigenous communities and acknowledge Indigenous peoples as the original inhabitants of ancestral lands.

In *Red Skin, White Masks,* Glenn Sean Coulthard asserts that the theory and practice of Indigenous anticolonialism "is best understood as a struggle primarily inspired by and oriented around *the question of land*—a struggle not only *for* land in the material sense, but also *deeply informed by what the land as a system of reciprocal relations and obligations* can teach us about living our lives in relation to one another and the natural world in nondominating and nonexploitative terms."[42] Land restitution, (Land Back) then, can be seen as the fundamental step for decolonization and returning to ancestral ways of living that are place-based and in reciprocal relationship with and kinship to the land that Indigenous peoples steward.

DECOLONIZATION

Decolonization and "the equitable distribution of land" is simultaneously about Native sovereignty, self-determination, and rights; and about the Earth and its resources being sustained, cared for, and lived with symbiotically. Colonization disrupted the communal responsibility to land inherent in Indigenous nationhood, and turned land into a private commodity for wealth extraction and accumulation. Therefore, a decolonial lens of returning land to Indigenous nations, not just individuals, is necessary to avoid reproducing those dynamics.[43]

The colonial matrix of power, coined by Peruvian sociologist and humanist thinker Anibal Quijano, refers to the neoliberal enmeshment of states and corporations in which "corporate entities and states are indistinguishable in their economic interests and activities; states act on behalf of corporations, and corporate entities hire security forces to control and suppress anti-extractivist organizing."[44]

Decolonization is the active process of resisting, transforming, and reclaiming imposed colonial structures through (re)asserting Indigenous lifeways and practicing Indigenous autonomy, sovereignty, and self-determination. Bonaventure Soh Bejeng Ndikung writes: "Decolonization is a way of being, existing and surviving that is underlined, framed and led by resistances, reclamations, restitutions, repatriations and reformations that are informed by a history of violence, dispossession and oppression. These topics are not comfortable. They are an affront and indignation towards colonization and coloniality and all the by-products of the colonial matrix of power."[45] Decolonization holds Indigenous sovereignty and self-determination of land (rematriation of land), resources, and cultural, political, and economic systems at the center.

During the 1940s–1960s, the term *decolonization* referred to revolutionary movements across Africa gaining countries political independence and autonomy from colonial rule.

The largest and most successful widespread revolt against colonial rule took place in Haiti from 1791 to 1804. The enslaved people of Haiti fought and won their independence from France and became the first free Black republic in the world and the first nation to permanently ban slavery. Reporter Greg Rosalsky writes, "It was an independent, black-led nation—created by slaves who had cast aside their chains and fought their oppressors for their freedom—during a time when white-led nations were enforcing brutal, racist systems of exploitation around the world."

In the aftermath, under continued threats of violence and takeover, Haiti was coerced into paying France 150 million francs to maintain their independence in what has been called "The Greatest Heist in History."[46] According to National Public Radio, "The amount was too much for the young nation to pay outright, and so it had to take out loans with hefty interest rates from a French bank. Over the next century, Haiti paid French slaveholders and their descendants the equivalent of between \$20 and \$30 billion in today's dollars. It took Haiti 122 years to pay it off."[47]

The 1945 Pan-African Congress demanded independence of African nations, with those in attendance including leaders and thinkers such as Kwame Nkrumah, Jomo Kenyatta, Dr. W.E.B. DuBois, Hastings Banda, and Amy Garvey. "We believe in the rights of all peoples to govern themselves. We affirm the right of all colonial peoples to control their own destiny. All colonies must be free from foreign imperialist control, whether political or economic," Nkrumah wrote in a declaration from the 1945 Congress. He went on to lead the independence movement of Ghana, the first sub-Saharan African nation to achieve independence, autonomy, and political decolonization from European control in 1957. Frantz Fanon's influential 1961 text on decolonization, *The Wretched of the Earth*, explicitly states that decolonization will require a "change in the order of the world."

The meaning of decolonization has become diluted as it has become popularized, hashtagged, and commercialized in online and academic spaces. Decolonization as a metaphor, as in the phrase "decolonizing one's mind" or decolonizing a specific field of study, subsumes the goals of decolonization into the aims of other projects for social justice. This rhetorical use of the word *decolonization* lacks the bottom line of centering the material nature that decolonization calls for. Eve Tuck and K. Wayne Yang offer a clear understanding of what

decolonization is *not:* "It is not converting Indigenous politics to a Western doctrine of liberation; it is not a philanthropic process of 'helping' the at-risk and
alleviating suffering; it is not a generic term for struggle against oppressive conditions and outcomes. . . . Decolonization is not a metonym for social justice."[48]

Decolonization calls for deconstructing and dismantling settler-colonial systems, which fundamentally and specifically involves land restitution, Indigenous
political self-determination and governance of resources, and securing sovereign Indigenous futures.

REFLECTIONS ON HISTORY AND CEREMONY
For All of Us

We've covered a lot of ground in this chapter. Let's take a breath. Take a moment
to check in: how are you doing with all of this? It is impossible to absorb so much
information and the weight of its meaning in one sitting. This might be a good time
to take a break. Know that you can come back to this as many times as you need.
This is a starting point, and unlearning colonial culture is a lifelong process.

Getting to know the medicines we are engaging with requires getting to
know their place in a human, historical, and biocultural context. There needs to
be space to process the discomfort, guilt, shame, confusion, and other difficult
emotions that are natural responses to the horrors that have taken place. Healing
can only extend as far as we are willing to clean out the wounds.

Spend some time sitting with and seeking to understand the history of events
that have led to this current moment in psychedelics. These medicines have been
loved, stolen, outlawed, removed from their homes, dissected, embraced in new
contexts, and turned into global commodities. I wonder, do we ever ask them how
they are faring in all of this? What tending they need? What does this suggestion
bring up for you? Getting to know a medicine can be like getting to know someone
who is going to be important in your life. Take the time to be curious, listen, and sit
with the nuances and difficulties of what you might uncover.

All of us now benefiting from the psychedelic resurgence must also grapple
with the impacts of the drug war. Beyond advocating for the medicines we love, it
is crucial that we leverage this public attention to drive action against the ongoing
drug war fueling the Prison-Industrial Complex. A few questions to consider:

- What is the distinction (if any) between drugs, psychedelics, and plant
  medicines? How attached am I to these beliefs? How do I relate to people
  who see this differently?

- What was I taught about drugs and the people who use them? Who did
  I learn this from?

- What parts of this chapter challenged me or brought up discomfort? Why might that be?

- What misconceptions have I had about Indigenous communities?

- What is my relationship with the Indigenous communities who originally made their homes in the place where I now live? Where can I learn more about their history and their present-day lived realities?

- How has the drug war touched my life or the lives of people I love? How has it touched other communities I am not a part of?

- What can I do to contribute to healing and repair for communities harmed by colonization and the drug war?

For Journeyers

Sit with your personal and cultural history to understand how you make sense of your life events and the ancestral events in your lineage that have shaped the life you are currently experiencing. This takes time and is best done from a place of curiosity and observation. If we attach our identities too tightly to our personal and ancestral histories, we can risk running into defensiveness, collapse, or overwhelm. We don't have to solve the problems of the world or shoulder the weight of healing our entire ancestral lines. We can view the process of coming into understanding as a gift.

Your personal history will affect your needs and experiences as you go about medicine work. Generally, the more you can build awareness of what you are carrying with you, the more fruitful and clarifying your journeys will be.

For Facilitators

Explore your personal and cultural history and the way it affects your philosophy, vulnerabilities, and approach to the work. Relating to inner-work, become intimately familiar with your own ancestral line and the medicines that were a part of your lineage in past generations. Spend time unpacking what it means to participate in medicines from other lineages, and how to reconcile this participation. Think seriously about whether you have permission to serve the medicines you serve, and how the medicine and its people may be impacted by this choice.

Before working with a new client, spend time sharing what you have learned about the roots of this medicine and the people who have stewarded it. Get comfortable naming and acknowledging difficult questions around Indigenous use, permission, and reciprocity. Develop a practice around continuous learning and engaging around the histories of these medicines. It is impossible to be an expert of your chosen medicine; maintain a learner's mind as the years pass. Seek out mentorship from culture bearers who can provide added context. Spend time listening to elders and understand how and why certain medicine customs were shaped and why ceremonies are conducted in particular ways. Allow this foundation of history to be a catalyst for practices of reciprocity, in both life and medicine work.

In Conversation with Kwasi Adusei, DNP

In spite of growing enthusiasm and promising policy efforts, the use of these mind-altering substances is illegal in most places. While in some cases they hold less of a law enforcement priority or lower penalties compared to other more marginalized substances, there are still real risks associated with growing, possessing, using, or distributing these substances. The risks are compounded for people who are racialized or experience marginalization due to immigration, socioeconomic status, and other factors. I spoke with my dear friend and colleague, Dr. Kwasi Adusei, about the world of mental health, psychedelics, and community organizing toward collective change.

Dr. Kwasi Adusei is a Ghanaian psychiatric mental health nurse practitioner and the founder of the Psychedelic Society of Western New York, from which he developed a local psychedelic harm-reduction organization. Kwasi is also a trainee of the MAPS-sponsored MDMA-assisted psychotherapy for PTSD and was part of the initial therapists of color cohort.

In addition to being a psychiatric nurse practitioner who works in community mental health and a leading voice in social justice in the psychedelic field, Kwasi has experienced the impacts of the drug war firsthand. During a traffic stop on his way to provide harm-reduction services at a festival in 2017, Kwasi was arrested for possession of psilocybin mushrooms. Kwasi knows firsthand how detrimental an encounter with the police and prison system can be. He was fortunate enough to avoid incarceration through a prison diversion program, but faced immediate and lasting impacts due to the arrest. Fortunately, Kwasi remains a community leader in the psychedelic field, much to our collective benefit.

Psychedelic advocates need to be aware that these events are continuing to happen. Our work is not finished, with destigmatization and widespread access. The risks of possession are still very real, and they disproportionately harm communities of color. As powerful and beautiful as these medicines are, we cannot get too comfortable to remember we are in a climate of prohibition, criminalization, and rising policy brutality and immunity that is literally life-threatening for some of our community members.

RM: *I would love to hear about what brought you to this work originally, and why you find it compelling as a part of your path.*

KA: Like so many of us, what brought me to this work originally was a personal experience. I had many experiences that in some way, shape, or form, compounded and led to transformative shifts in the way that I looked at the world and myself. I work with ketamine in my current practice as a DNP. And I continue to meet with people in whom I see so much of myself or my potential selves. Every moment, we are starting from this place of potential. At any point in our lives. And there are so many things that can happen that can lead us in one direction or another.

But nonetheless, certain experiences really shifted my perspective, my relationship with myself and the circumstances of my life. I worked in community mental health for a fair bit of time. I witnessed a lot of trauma, and really ran up against the moral injury and the sense of hopelessness. I started to recognize how corrupt and maladaptive many systems are.

RM: *Can you say more about that?*

KA: If we're talking about history, we can look at how every system that exists now was created with an intention and a purpose. And so what we see is always a function of that initial intention and purpose. And so having worked in the mental health system, I saw firsthand that it's kind of a bad investment. We are pouring all of this money into something that's not working. We're starting to realize that the mental health system doesn't really exist to help people. It just exists to maintain the bottom. It helps some people from falling through the cracks. It's preventing suicide and a lot of the more severe social ills, but really, it's not there to heal. So the premise mental health is built upon is not about thriving or systemic repair, it's about mitigating risks and worst-case scenarios.

So I entered a field with that being a driver in many capacities. Not only this, but it's a system that was draining me, that I was sacrificing parts of my soul in order to participate in it. And I was surrounded by all these people within that system who were only wanting to do good and support people. That experience really just helped to justify and clarify that something needed to be different. Psychedelics seemed really promising because I've seen personal benefit from it. But there is also something deeper, about the psychedelics not necessarily being here only for healing the individual.

What I was most curious about was how psychedelics can change the systems that we have. So now it's not just about healing people. Beyond that, what are we learning and integrating, in the work that we're providing? How can we really start asking deeper questions about disconnection and why people are sick? Questions that can help us expand our perspective and look at the ways the ills of society are leading to the ills of the individual.

RM: *We're coming out of a fifty-year drug war. In your view, how can we move forward in a way that's balanced?*

KA: It's important that we offer a balanced perspective for people. It's already a struggle, even before widespread decriminalization. Lots of ketamine clinics are experiencing this, where a client has one session with ketamine, and says, "I'm not completely cured." And they're upset. It's not their fault. It's because of how their expectations have been set up.

The narrative around psychedelics is changing constantly. For a period of time, it was for fun. For a period of time, it was for self-exploration. Now, for a period of time, it is for mental health and wellness. Do you see what I mean?

Beyond this, the next period of time will likely be rooted in spirituality. I see that as the next piece of the arc. Even with a spiritual emergence, going through these spiritual experiences, it's a very messy process, but people are really only looking at it from the perspective of healing, which is often attached to a predefined outcome. The framing defines the experience. If someone sets out to have a spiritual experience with its own timeline and life cycle, their sense of how it is unfolding will look different than if someone is trying to alleviate specific symptoms.

In my work, psychiatry, you have to be very cautious about the kind of conversations that you're having. Everything has to be evidence based. So people only have the perspective of, "Is this going to heal my wounds?"

There are practices that can be supported by and supportive of the psychedelic experiences. We don't have to have psychedelics as the anchor. And so what are the accessible anchors that we can start working on? I believe mindfulness practices need to begin well before the psychedelic experiences are happening.

A lot of our responsibility as professionals in this field is getting people adequately prepared before they dive into the medicine, which I think is another one of the shifts like another one of the vectors from the way that we do things in mental healthcare generally. Of course, integration is important. Of course, it's where you have the capacity to integrate insights into your life and integrate yourself into the world. But I don't think we have enough of a focus on the preparation experiences.

RM: *It feels like preparation is the next major edge of the public conversation— really looking into and unpacking the way our daily habits can help increase the possibility that psychedelic experiences can seed lasting shifts in a person's life. That the benefits will stick or take hold, so to speak. And resourcing people to begin or deepen those daily practices.*

KA: I often think about the culture and protocols surrounding ayahuasca, which is sacred medicine. Most people have been taught to hold it with a great deal of reverence. And there are protocols where you go into a ceremony with a *dieta,* being very intentional to honor the forms of fasting that are required— not just an edible fast, but a spiritual fast.

We don't think in the same way about other tools of spirit, like psilocybin, or man-made tools that connect us to spirit, like LSD or ketamine. We don't think or talk nearly as much about preparation diets or spiritual diets—I wonder, could we learn from the way that we treat ayahuasca and apply those principles of reverence and preparation across the psychedelic landscape?

RM: *I'd love to hear you speak, as a clinician and a community organizer, about your perspective on policy change priorities.*

KA: I think clinical care and community access certainly complement each other. But decriminalization needs to come first. Across the board. Whether it's psilocybin or any modality that people are using to find some healing, we have to decriminalize it before we talk about medicalizing and legalizing.

When people are seeking out medicines that are criminalized, they are facing a serious legal risk. And we are partially responsible for that narrative, as participants in this field and advocates for public access. The true harms of this medicine are the law, prohibition. So I think for that reason alone, it's more than enough reason to justify that decriminalization needs to come first.

Many of us have to sit with the tension of being between worlds. For me, part of the tension is knowing that some of the things I say and dream could put my license at risk. I sit with that on a daily basis. What happens to those of us who could lose our licenses? There's something about the need for community-based healing and support that is core to my values system.

Really, it's all about having many points of access. It's not correct to say that medicalization is going to restrict access. It will create *some* access. It's just an incomplete picture. There are a lot of people who won't have access at all unless there is a medical path for them. But community-based access is key. Because if people just don't have access to these kinds of healing practices and knowledge in their backyards with the people they trust, and if we have laws that prevent community-based medicine, but allow corporations and companies to be the holders of such a precious resource . . . that's really just going to continue serving the attainment of wealth for a few as opposed to feeding true community wellness. There is an element of radical reliance that a community can have on itself, and that is a healthy thing; that is where the energy needs to be just from a societal standpoint.

RM: *Right, exactly. Community participation is one of the beautiful things that has come out of the underground due to existing on the margins. How do you see social action playing a role in integration?*

KA: Integration should include social change in some capacity. But there is really this natural element of allowing the overflow of our healing to pour into the benefit of all mankind in various capacities. And I sort of see it as this really beautiful breath, you know, so there's an inhale, which is that support, that soothing that you need for your mind, for your body, for your soul that you need to do for yourself, filling your cups. And then there's the exhale, it doesn't go without the exhale, right, and you can't have one without the other.

I believe that following that path, creates that, you know, multidimensional reconnection to nature, community, self, others, so on and so forth. That might go missing because we're so focused on just healing ourselves and healing ourselves and healing ourselves. This reconnection is such a natural thing that wants to happen. People just don't have clarity and it's not spoken about as much. But I believe it's quite clear that once we have the language to describe processes, it starts to click. It's no longer an unspoken knowing and everything starts opening up, and structures start changing. We start thinking a lot differently and more expansively about what programming can look like, what integration can look like. So I think it's a really interesting piece that I'd really love to see us leaning more into.

RM: *Everything changes when we see participation in community healing as the natural outpouring of our own healing. I believe that is the nature of reciprocity. When I am healing, I don't want to hoard the goodness for myself; I want to share it. What's possible and that we not only can change but we are changing, you know, and that there is this inner healer in the broadest sense moving us in the direction of justice, wholeness, and reconciliation.*

Conclusion

Coming to terms with our individual and collective history can be an overwhelming process. There are many generations of wounds and beauty to uncover, and it is common during psychedelic journeys to access not only one's own biographical material, but also that of past generations and more broadly, what some refer to as the collective unconscious. This is work we must hold together.

We must also remember that the forces of colonialism cannot be attributed to a single person or group of people. It is a societal sickness that has spanned many generations and wrapped itself around the globe. Because there is such a charge to these topics, we need to resource ourselves with tools to manage what comes up. Notice the resistance, shame, grief, and moral injury that arise. Ask the medicines for help. Remember that bearing witness to our shared history doesn't equate to accepting the blame for the project of colonization or the violence of the drug war. These are forces we all unknowingly participate in due to conditioning. Acknowledgment of our shared history opens up the possibility to move through it and begin to heal it.

History is at the heart of everything we are doing in this field; we are dealing with history and we are shaping it. The capacity for healing is only as great as our capacity to acknowledge what has occurred, be present with the downstream impacts of those events, and return to more generative ways to live as we move forward. The more we create space for truth and reconciliation, the more possibility we open up for writing new histories in our lifetimes.

CHAPTER 12

Reciprocity

Note: *This chapter is coauthored by Juliette Mohr.*

Introduction

Nature exists in a dynamic balance of interconnected relationships and exchanges. When more is taken than returned, the results are depletion, imbalance, and system collapse. Many people in the Global North have the advantage of enjoying psychedelics simply by purchasing them or receiving them as a gift. Most of the psychedelic field is no longer in direct connection with the medicines' roots or required to know where they came from, who grew them, or how they were sourced and produced. The current psychedelic field does not bear the historic or contemporary burdens carried by those for whom entheogens are integral to their way of life.

The psychedelic movement is surging, in part because many of us have had the privilege of accessing direct, life-altering experiences with these substances. These medicines, whether grown or synthesized, give generously—often in the form of healing, wonder, reconnection, play, and illumination. But they don't exist in a vacuum; they come from beautiful and specific historic and biocultural contexts. Thankfully, these sacraments also support the capacity for openness—and this unlocks a door to a more nuanced and responsible conversation about where our medicines come from, their historical/cultural lineage, and the impacts of our participation in what has become, for better or worse, a global market.

Just as being good stewards on this earth requires us to know the stories behind our food, clothing, fuel, and devices—among other things—we also have a responsibility to ask deeper questions about psychedelics. What do we *not* know about the places, cultures, ecologies, peoples, and complex histories associated with the healing modalities we venerate? Why might that be? In asking these questions, we can uncover practical and meaningful ways to contribute to a culture of reciprocity, sustainability, and integrity toward the benefit of all. Then we can begin to see the ways reciprocity lays the groundwork for collective healing.

Sacred reciprocity is an integral step in the process of relationship building, showing up, and practicing accountability in psychedelics. While it is not possible to erase the harm that occurred or ignore the power dynamics embedded in the field as it stands, we do have an opportunity, and responsibility, to course-correct and disrupt the imbalanced, extractive ways of being that have brought us this far.

Shifting to Reciprocity

As has been discussed throughout this book, healing is not possible until we take time to examine the wounds we need to heal. This is precisely why healing can be so uncomfortable. The Western fantasy of individualism is just that: a fantasy. The laws of the natural world and wisdom of Indigenous peoples demonstrate plainly that we are deeply interconnected. The wounds of colonial violence affect us all, whether we are descendants of colonized peoples, settlers, or a blend of both. While we have different roles to play, it is imperative that we take steps to heal this history. Fortunately, we have been blessed with plant allies that help us along the way. In this way, the site of the wound also holds the medicine.

We are living in a period of collective awakening and the continued pursuit of racial justice and Indigenous sovereignty, which are essential for humanity to heal. In reaction to these movements, there has also emerged a resistance within the psychedelic field from people who seem to believe they are color-blind, we are all one, or we should not dwell on the painful truths of the past. There is an impulse to move on from true events and an intolerance for the ugliness of our shared history.

Spiritual bypassing and shutting down discourse are manifestations of a desire to look the other way. I have personally interacted in private and public forums with colleagues who become fragile or even aggressive when the topics of reciprocity, land, and Indigenous sovereignty arose (no matter how compassionately the conversation was approached). This is a cause for concern.

It is painful to acknowledge the atrocities that laid the path for the modern "psychedelic renaissance." To come to terms with the violence that has occurred toward Indigenous peoples around the world is to have your heart broken. To consider that we are also beneficiaries of this violence is to experience moral injury. And yet, there is no way forward but through. When we confront the impacts of colonialism and begin to see how they show up as harms in our communities, organizations, and personal lives, we can begin to change. Again, awareness opens up new possibilities.

So, consider this an invitation. As we spend some time going deeper into the implications of our shared history, we can take an opportunity to get curious about our own edges. We can take breaks and come back. We can have brave, difficult conversations and messy, imperfect exchanges without stepping on anyone else's dignity or humanity. It's okay to fumble through. We can practice the very things we hope to find more of in the world—tenderness, courage, compassion, repair.

It is my hope that the global network of psychedelic communities will recognize that the struggle for Indigenous sovereignty is not only a step closer to right relationship with the medicines we love, it is also good for everyone. The thriving of Indigenous peoples means an honoring of our shared humanity, the thriving of ecosystems, the preservation of sacred medicines, and the opportunity to seed new possibilities beyond the legacies of violence and domination. That is a world I want to live in.

Defining Reciprocity

Reciprocity is more than a benefit-sharing model, or sending a percentage of profits to Indigenous projects. Reciprocity as a relational dynamic should reflect the values of the person, plant, or group we are seeking reciprocity with—or else it is not truly reciprocal. If reciprocity is meant to establish and maintain right relationship with Indigenous communities, it is important to act through a shared understanding of reciprocity that aligns with Indigenous cultures' conceptions of what reciprocity means, looks like, and feels like.

TRANSACTIONAL RECIPROCITY

Western notions view reciprocity as a transactional relationship of benefit-sharing. This orientation of reciprocity more closely resembles charity or philanthropy, where one party is a benefactor and the other party is a beneficiary. This dynamic of reciprocity is troubling, as it can serve to further maintain and uphold imbalances of power through "giving back" to a community that has been the recipient of exploitation and extraction. Transactional reciprocity is not truly collaborative as it does not analyze and challenge dynamics of power, and the terms of the arrangement are defined by the benefactor. Fulfilling only the bare minimum of what a reciprocal relationship entails, the dynamic can come across as paternalistic or charitable, and often stems from white saviorism, guilt, obligation due to public pressure, or a desire for favorable optics.

North American Indigenous researcher LaDonna Harris and coauthor Jacqueline Wasilewski caution against reciprocity that reinforces imbalances of power, writing that Indigenous conceptions of reciprocity "should never,

ever, even have a hint of superiority or imposition. . . . 'Charity' creates a status difference between giver and receiver, with the giver in the higher position. Creating such a status difference devalues the gift."[1] This is an example of how transactional benefit-sharing models of reciprocity communicate a lack of cultural competence, fail to take power dynamics into account, and miss the opportunity to engage with Indigenous conceptions of reciprocity in a way that can build lasting relationships based on respect. Given the wider climate of extraction, exclusion, abuse on all levels, and the delegitimization and deval-uation of Indigenous knowledge within the psychedelic space, it is important to question intentions behind efforts for sacred reciprocity, and work to make sure the impact of an approach is truly aligned with the intention of reciprocity. Especially with regard to reciprocity projects, it is important to "come cor-rect" when engaging with Indigenous peoples.[2] Reciprocity with this in mind cannot simply seek to give back, but must spring forth from a sense of respon-sibility to cultivate relationships of repair and make sure these communities are receiving their fair due in a way that is fitting and appropriate for them, on their terms.

SACRED RECIPROCITY

Sacred reciprocity is the heartfelt exchange, gratitude, and acknowledgment for everyone and everything that sustains us. In psychedelics, it is a call for those who consume plant medicines to give back and serve meaningfully to the com-munities and lineages who have preserved these medicines for generations. Indigenous communities bear the impact of the expansion, along with, in many cases, oppression from local governments.

The concept of sacred reciprocity comes from the Quechua word *ayni*. Quechua is the Indigenous language of the ancestral peoples of the Andes, spe-cifically Peru. *Ayni* is a principle of receptivity and gratitude, marked by a life-style of giving back in an inhale-exhale type relationship with the natural world, thus holding our place in life's cycles with dynamic balance.

Even those who consume only lab-based substances can participate in sacred reciprocity through a number of the practices detailed in this chapter. In this way, reciprocity is an act of integration, a way of weaving in and paying for-ward the benefits we have received from these powerful substances. It is a way of establishing right relationship, which is foundational to deep healing.

DEEP RECIPROCITY

Deep reciprocity is a way of living. It moves beyond medicine and into how we experience ourselves and the world on a daily basis. Deep reciprocity is justice work. Focused on mutual transformation, it holds themes of relationality, inter-connectedness, and the iterative nature of generative cycles within the web that holds us. Author Leanne Simpson asserts that responsibility and reciprocity are an alternative to a colonial extractivist mindset:

> When people extract things, they're taking and they're running and they're using it for just their own good. What's missing is the respon-sibility. If you're not developing relationships with the people, you're not giving back, you're not sticking around to see the impact of the extraction. You're moving to someplace else. The alternative is deep reciprocity. It's respect, it's relationship, it's responsibility, and it's local. If you're forced to stay in your 50-mile radius, then you very much are going to experience the impacts of extractivist behavior.[3]

Deep reciprocity centers a perspective that values and respects Indigenous voices, is grounded in the context of power dynamics, and creates opportunities for collaboration and open sharing of knowledge—encouraging all parties to grow and support one another's growth. A deep, generativity-oriented reciprocity—which can be found not only in Indigenous and non-Western knowledge systems, but also within disciplines of ecology, systems thinking, quantum physics, and chaos theory—goes beyond the normative sense of rela-tionality into a deeper understanding of a world where all beings and know-ledges exist within web-like networks of relationship.

Deep reciprocity includes an active and deliberate analysis of power, privi-lege, and oppression, providing transformative potential within engaged parties, systems, and paradigms.[4] Deep reciprocity is generative; it leverages transfor-mational synergies emerging from deep, relational, conscious expressions of reciprocity to impact and shape not only what entities do, but how entities are. In other words, to walk in deep reciprocity is to consent to being changed by relationship.

Harris and Wasilewski describe four core values commonly found within North American Indigenous tribes that traverse generation, geography, and tribe. These principles are also known as the Four R's: Relationship, Responsibility, Reciprocity, and Redistribution. According to Harris and Wasilewski, Indigenous conceptions of reciprocity are understood as *cyclical obligation*, referring to Indig-enous notions of time, relationships, and nature as circular instead of linear. The authors write that "the Indigenous idea of reciprocity is based on very long rela-tional dynamics in which we are all seen as 'kin' to each other."[5]

Reciprocity goes hand in hand with redistribution (the *sharing obligation*), which works to balance and rebalance uneven dynamics. Sacred reciprocity within the psychedelic ecosystem should move beyond transaction to align more closely with a deep paradigm of reciprocity. This would mean that systems of power and oppression are considered and reciprocity becomes an expression of giving and receiving within an engaged, relational, and transformative perspective.

Further, we need to be aware that working toward right relationship is not a cure-all that will magically erase the harms of the past or restore balance to current power structures. Eduardo Schenberg considers, "Neither the type of financial compensation provided by a benefit-sharing contract, nor a research project approved by Indigenous peoples, can address the harm done by epistemic injustices and unfair regulatory models that do not contemplate traditional medicine." Epistemic injustice is defined by Miranda Fricker as an injustice in which a group is determined to be incapable of making sense and meaning of their own experiences.[6]

Sacred reciprocity built on the foundation of creating transformative relationships of care and supporting Indigenous communities on their own terms can illuminate the path forward in a time of mainstreaming psychedelic plant medicines. This idea follows traditional conceptions of the ayahuasca journey within Huni Kuin cosmology, in which the *Nixi Pae* drinker participates in the "continuous metamorphosis which relates to the transformation principle, the primordial creation."[7] We transform our deeper systems and are transformed ourselves by *walking with* one another on this journey together, in ways that value one another and our multiplicity. The conversation about reciprocity changes when we shift our understanding of our lives, work, and identities from a framework of transaction to one of relationship. It shifts from a practice of obligation to one of belonging. The togetherness expressed through reciprocity is central to our personal and collective healing.

Exploring Reciprocity

SPIRITUAL VIOLENCE

Spiritual abuse is defined as actions that damage a person or community's subjective experience and practice of the sacred, potentially harming the spiritual integrity and spiritual resources for an entire community.[8] Linda Tuhiwai Smith's work conceptualizes extraction as operating through the conversion of *Indigeneity* into exchange value.[9] This has been done to all forms of Indigeneity, but an overlooked component is the richness of Indigenous spiritual resources.

In her paper, "Lost Saints: Desacralization, Spiritual Abuse and Magic Mushrooms," Anna Lutkajtis examines the impacts of the West's psilocybin discovery and popularity on the Mazatec community, arguing that the misappropriation of Indigenous sacred practices has resulted in the desacralization of psilocybin mushrooms, constituting a form of spiritual abuse with extensive and lasting harmful consequences. Desacralization is defined as the "reverse of sacralization, and occurs when a formerly dedicated sacred object is used for another purpose outside of the particular religious setting which dedicated it for a sacred purpose, hence rendering the object desacralized."[10] Considering the aftermath of R. Gordon Wasson's initial encounter with psilocybin mushrooms, including a hippie frenzy in Huautla de Jiménez that resulted in a long-term police presence, the negative consequences impacting María Sabina in her later life, and the ultimate form of desacralization—the worldwide classification of *the little saints* as illicit drugs—Lutkajtis maintains that the spiritual power of psilocybin mushrooms has been contaminated, thereby stripped from those who have practiced with them for centuries.[11]

Commercialization of the mushroom *velada* ceremonies has also contributed to the desacralization of the *velada* as well as the reputation of Huasteco healers and healing practices—all of which constitute spiritual abuse. Apolonio Teran, a Mazatec healer contemporary of María Sabina, claimed in an interview with Alvaro Estrada that "the divine mushroom no longer belongs to us. Its sacred language has been profaned. The language has been spoiled and it is indecipherable for us. . . .The mushrooms have a divine spirit: They always had it for us, but the foreigners arrived and frightened it away."[12] The diminished force, or spiritual integrity, of the mushrooms due to commercialization, contamination, appropriation, and prohibition are all examples of spiritual abuse.

These experiences have created lasting harm to the community of Huautla de Jiménez on a deeply spiritual and emotional level. Today, Huautla is still negatively impacted by Western associations of psilocybin mushrooms and María Sabina's image in a way that has been damaging for the community and degrading to the reputation of its Mazatec healers. Duke and Faudree's work on the Huautla community denotes a sense of distress and loss due to the cultural degradation of the mushroom *velada,* while Flores explains from a Mazatec perspective the essential need for acknowledgment of the legacy of violence that has characterized the experiences of the Mazatec community post-Wasson.[13]

What does sacred reciprocity mean in a greater set and setting of material, intellectual, and spiritual extraction and abuse? Where does sacred reciprocity come into play with substances that have been desacralized for the original users of these plants? As we discuss reciprocity, we have to hold the tension of many things being true at once: the destruction that has occurred within communities as these medicines have been globalized, and the incredible benefits many of us now experience thanks to their globalization. I would not be writing this book if not for the spread of the psilocybin mushroom *veladas* beyond Mexico. We can hold these truths with compassion while also committing to not repeat the same cycles of harm.

SCIENCE AND INDIGENOUS KNOWLEDGE

Colonialism shaped dominant epistemologies and narratives, centering modern scientific knowledge over folk knowledge, and favoring centralized, institutionalized ways of knowing nature over localized, informal ways of relating to it.[14] In many ways, the "psychedelic renaissance" is often centered around modern science "confirming" what Indigenous knowledge systems have known for centuries.

For example, biomedical research with psychedelics has increasingly caught on to the value of spiritual or mystical experiences as a key factor in growth, healing, meaning-making, and reducing symptoms of emotional distress. Importantly, these were precisely the aspects of Indigenous psychedelic shamanism so often cast aside as primitive, unscientific superstitious beliefs, again enacting the cycle of epistemic injustices highlighted by Eduardo Schenberg.[15]

A parallel to this process can be seen with the ideologies held by the Mexican scientific and medical community upon discovering Indigenous and folk healing uses of peyote in the early 1900s. The Huichol people during this time were cast as the noble savage, knowledgeable about peyote as a plant but lacking in "proper" understanding of the drug, as a result of their perceived separateness from Western civilization and modernity. The Instituto Médico Nacional (IMN) in Mexico took great interest in researching the potential therapeutic properties of peyote, believing it had real power and effect. As Alexander Dawson writes, that power simply needed to be "harnessed properly, in a way that discarded the delusions and superstitions of the Indians for a modern, scientific approach to the cactus."[16] The same colonial mindset of epistemic injustices occurring in the early 1900s is being reproduced a century later within the discourse of Western psychedelic science and therapeutic applications.

Ideologically, the practice of scientific research and data has a few impacts: It distances psychedelics from the Indigenous communities and knowledge systems from which they originated and transforms psychedelic plants into isolated compounds through Western technological means. It also seeks to sequester and own these compounds as intellectual property through patenting and uses Western knowledge production to advance novel pharmaceutical uses of these compounds in a codified, controlled Western context.

As Leanne Simpson explains, "The extractivist mindset isn't about having a conversation and having a dialogue and bringing in Indigenous knowledge on the terms of Indigenous peoples. It is very much about extracting whatever ideas scientists . . . thought were good and assimilating it."[17] Science is the language through which Indigenous knowledge is assimilated into a Western view of legitimacy. With assimilation, Indigenous knowledge is incorporated into a dominant culture by reshaping and decontextualizing the knowledge from wider Indigenous cultural contexts, then reframing the knowledge into "new" scientific breakthroughs. We must consider what one calls "new" and for whom it is so, concerned that Western psychology and medicine's psychedelic revolution involves a "delicate exercise of becoming legitimate, of building an evidence-based regime and validating within the hegemonic science, new—well, actually very old treatments."[18]

These practices of extraction and assimilation are enacted when Western scientists and researchers come to the Sierra Mazateca and patronize Mazatec *chjota chijne* (wisdom bearers) by stating that they incorrectly call their own mushrooms by the wrong name and are mistaken about the range of their local mushrooms.[19] Ayahuasca Maestra Vicky Corisepa comments on this experience, sharing that "[the foreigners] say things like, *'these native people are a bunch of ignorants, they know nothing,'* without recognizing that we're the first that mastered the medicine. They've taken the knowledge from us, the foreigners with their financial power."[20]

The colonial view of psychedelic plant medicines invalidates Indigenous knowledge by relegating Indigenous knowledge (and peoples) to the past. In "Native Liberation: The Way Forward," Nick Estes writes that "natives are thought to be a backwards people living in the past."[21] For example, while María Sabina died in 1985—only eleven years before Timothy Leary—she is depicted as a representation of something and somewhere ancient and devoid of modernity, someone only to be interacted with in ethnographic study, not as a contemporary or taken with intellectual sincerity.

How can traditional practice and Indigenous ways of knowing coexist in the coming years? We must begin by recognizing the imbalanced relationship they currently have.

Not all forms of research are or have to be extractive. There are growing movements to advance citizen-led, participatory action research projects. For example, in *Decolonizing Methodologies,* author and educator Linda Tuhiwai Smith lays out the historical background of research and colonialism and highlights that research can and should be designed to support people in improving their current conditions, while pointing to ethical research protocols held within Maori communities as guiding lights.[22]

Regardless of context, we must consider the following questions when setting out to attain knowledge:

- Who (people, communities, or institutions) is leading the project?
- Why is the research being done? What is the end goal?
- Whose knowledge is being utilized or pulled from?
- Who needs to be responsible, accountable, consulted, and informed of the project?
- Who ultimately benefits from the data gathered? (Individuals, companies, local communities, broad populations such as North American and European citizens benefiting from psychedelic research, creating pathways to access and treatments)
- What are the implications and downstream impacts of this data being disseminated at scale?

THE NATURAL COLONIAL GAZE FRAMEWORK

The Natural Colonial Gaze Framework[23] is a concept created by Juliette Mohr to better understand the lens through which the colonial mind sees nature. This framework provides a structure for tracing the ideological lineage of the separation of nature from culture. It identifies colonial thought and encounter as the key agent in disseminating and enforcing an extractive way of engaging with the natural world. In our current times, around much of this planet, the Natural Colonial Framework has spread as the dominant way of relating to nature. The colonizing mind looks at an ecosystem and sees resources rather than life; it sees raw material to be extracted rather than family. When the colonial mind looks at the ocean, it does not see magic and the endless ineffability; it sees dollar signs and profit waiting to be maximized.

James Baldwin once expressed this well: "There is reason, after all, that some people wish to colonize the moon, and others dance before it as an ancient friend." From this vantage point, nature is not something humans are a part of, but something separate from ourselves, something to be harnessed, dominated, controlled, and extracted from. Macarena Gómez-Barris, author of *The Extractive Zone: Social Ecologies and Decolonial Perspectives,* defines *extractivism* as "the violence of colonial capitalism and its 'afterlives' in trying to convert life into commodities." *Extractive capitalism* refers to "an economic system of violence that participates in 'thefts, borrowings, and forced removals' in order to reorganize social life and the natural world."[24] As life is converted to commodities through resource extraction, the profits benefit those who do the extracting, and the costs of ecological degradation are carried largely by Indigenous peoples and subsistence-based communities in the Global South.

Through deconstructing the Natural Colonial Gaze as a dominant way of thinking about and engaging with the natural world, we can begin to create, imagine, and reconnect with alternative ways of relating and solutions that address environmental issues from a decolonial perspective, allowing us to highlight existing alternatives, what Gómez-Barris calls "submerged perspectives" that work to challenge, disrupt, and resist the Natural Colonial Gaze as it exists today.[25]

As we discuss in chapter 6, on Power, there is no way to separate our relationship to power from our relationship to the land and the natural world. They are shaped by one another. We cannot be power hungry and have a healthy, reciprocal relationship to nature. As we heal and reach toward right relationship with power, we heal our relationship to nature as well. And as we recognize that humans *are* nature, our beliefs about humanity begin to shift. When this happens, we recognize that there are truly no "others"—that the beauty and dignity of all beings, and the grace of Indigenous peoples of the world, are a gift. This causes those of us from nations with a history of colonialism to reconsider hierarchical beliefs about the world.

The project of colonization was key in separating humans from nature, as it had already separated humans from one another through gender, race, and class-based hierarchies. People of all ancestries have been impacted by the global project of colonization. Settler colonialism took place in Canada, the United States, South Africa, Algeria, Australia, Russia, and many other countries. Under settler colonialism, lands were not only claimed as part of an empire; they were invaded and occupied by settlers from the occupying nations. This occupation usually involved genocide; land theft; forced assimilation; and eradication of peoples' cultures, religions, and traditions.

These lands were occupied by force through a repeated system of coercion, extermination, erasure, and assimilation. While colonialism has expanded beyond the taking of land, we still see active colonialism as well as the lingering effects of colonial cultural imperialism in the languages, customs, and worldviews of former colonies.

Consider the English Imperial project that now exists as the British Commonwealth, with King Charles remaining the symbolic head of state in fourteen countries. This is not without resistance: Barbados and Antigua have referendums and Jamaica may cut ties by 2025. The death of Queen Elizabeth sparked global discourse about the history of colonization and called into question the legitimacy of the monarchy and the institution of colonialism itself.

How This Happened

In medieval times, most European cultures viewed themselves as integrated within nature, and daily life was marked by attunement to natural cycles and processes. This changed during the Enlightenment era, when ideals such as Cartesian dualism, rationality, science, and the expansion of the market economy fueled a radical uncoupling of the natural world from the cultural sphere. Raymond Murphy writes of this era: "Reason [and rationality] has enabled humanity to escape from nature and remake it" in order to achieve mastery and dominance over the natural world.[26] During this period, the rise of rationalism and dualist logic created binary distinctions that still affect us today, such as reason versus emotionality, thinking mind versus the mechanical body, and civilization versus savagery.

The ideal of rationality was and continues to be weaponized by the colonial mind against Indigenous peoples and their homelands, portraying Indigenous land as "unused, underused, or empty" spaces (terra nullius) in need of rational reorganization by settlers for "proper" use.[27] This logic continues to portray psychedelic plant medicines as underused substances with untapped potential of "proper" use by scientific and medical applications.

This Natural Colonial Gaze was then exported from Europe across the world through notions of development, progress, and modernity. The era of colonial expansion had devastating consequences on how nature was viewed, how Indigenous peoples were treated, and what colonial powers could do to make nature more productive and beneficial to colonial interests. Nature became a resource to be owned and extracted from or a "wilderness" to be researched, protected, or displayed. Once nature had been denigrated and established below the realm of humanity, the colonization of land, ecosystems, and people were made legitimate through the myth of terra nullius, or "land belonging to no one." The ideological mechanisms that license humans to exploit nature also justify the exploitation and subjugation of women and colonized peoples, and support supremacism of nation, gender, and race.

Legacy Burdens

Like all groups who have been oppressed, people with Indigenous ancestry (including those Indigenous to Africa who were captured and enslaved in the United States and elsewhere) bear the ancestral trauma of these events. Events do not happen in isolation and painful truths cannot be simply forgotten. Each generation is connected with the parents, grandparents, children, and grandchildren in an interwoven line across time. The traumas from violence and oppression also reveal the powers of resistance, resilience, and adaptive mechanisms. But these traumas live on in our bodies, nervous systems, individual and collective memories, family systems, community structures, and cultures.

Those of us with European ancestry have bloodlines that might not have been actively involved with the violence of settler colonialism, but were direct or indirect beneficiaries of this violence. We also hold the guilt, shame, and moral injury of the inhumanity that has occurred in our ancestry. We have an opportunity to participate in repair processes in our lifetimes and those that follow. Resmaa Menakem's framework of Somatic Abolitionism and his book *My Grandmother's Hands* unpack how these burdens live in our bodies and provide guidance on strategies for beginning to unwind them.[28]

Reciprocity in the Medicine Space
REFLECTIONS FOR ALL OF US

Harris and Wasilewski express the importance of engaging in true dialogue as a starting point for building community, valuing one another, and transforming relationships from an extractive paradigm to one of mutual respect and reciprocity. For the writers, true dialogue

> Involves, as poet Joy Harjo says, "A venturing out beyond [the world we already know] by listening, by learning."[29] Through caring enough for each other to engage in true dialogue we enable ourselves to be ourselves together. In fact, we can only be ourselves together. We can only be a "self" in community. We are simultaneously both autonomous and connected. There are no private truths. We have to let the realities of others into our conceptual and emotional spaces and vice versa.[30]

When we engage in true, honest, open, sometimes challenging conversation, we can begin to establish a deep reciprocity with the potential to transform not only what we do, but how *we can be.* The ability to bridge across difference is a collective process that requires all of our participation to transform our relationships and engage in solidarity to transform the systems we live in. For Indigenous peoples facing dispossession, extraction, biopiracy, epistemic injustices, cultural destruction, and desacralization with the proliferation and widening acceptance of psychedelics in the West, supporting and valuing them demands a reverence and accompaniment in efforts for decolonization, sovereignty, and autonomy.

Indigenous healers have recently been organizing toward these goals in the Amazon; the Shipibo Healers Union released two statements on the issues of spiritual extraction and globalization of Ayahuasca, titled the Yarinacocha

Declaration (2018) and the Pronouncement of the Shipibo-Konibo-Xetebo Nation on the Globalization of Ayahuasca (2019). In the Yarinacocha Declaration, the Shipibo Healers Union declared that Shipibo-Konibo-Xetebo healing and expertise in medicinal plants are fundamentally "anti-colonialist forms of practice and knowledge, able to resist, transform and reconfigure with every difficulty and threat," emphasizing that "the work of healing and the struggle toward self-determination are not separable. They must move forward on the same path."[31] In the 2019 Pronouncement of the Shipibo-Konibo-Xetebo Nation on the Globalization of Ayahuasca, the Shipibo Healers Union acknowledged "rampant abuse by outsiders of our sacred plants and of the ancestral knowledge of Amazonian Peoples," stating that they are "tired of seeing our knowledge and ancestral practices appropriated by a cannibalistic Western system."[32] Reciprocity with Indigenous plant medicine communities should heed these words and explicitly work in solidarity with Indigenous self-determination and derive from decolonial and anticolonial frameworks.

It is clear that the healing potential of psychedelic plant medicines alone will not be enough to repair the deep harm against Indigenous stewards, or enough to transform systems of oppression influencing the way Westerners relate to Indigenous communities, traditions, knowledge systems, *cosmovisiones,* and more-than-human kin. The path for healing calls for wholehearted engagement in the work to transform oppressive systems of colonial violence by walking with Indigenous communities, participating in efforts toward self-determination, and practicing deep, generative reciprocity in which we can make change and be changed ourselves.

INDIGENEITY

In her book *Braiding Sweetgrass,* Anishinaabe author and scientist Robin Wall Kimmerer speaks of "becoming Indigenous to place" and highlights the practices we can each participate in to restore our original relationship with the natural world. This is not to be mistaken as claiming Indigeneity for ourselves.

Note on Indigeneity: the concept of *Indigeneity* itself is complex and difficult to separate from colonial ideas such as blood quantum, a construct of the US federal government. By defining who was "legitimately" Native American by defining their percentage of Native blood, the government was able to use blood quantum policies to restrict the number of "legitimate card-carrying" Indians and, as a result, restrict Indigenous communities from holding the full measure of land promised to them. In addition, this harmed tribal members who did not meet blood quantum by reducing Indigeneity to bloodline and diminishing the cultural and relational aspects so central to Native life.

Perhaps readers have never considered the Indigenous roots of their own ancestral lines. Many of us have been long severed from our own family lines or can only trace a few generations back, through a period that was marked by the colonial project. While it is true that technically, if you trace it back far enough, we are all Indigenous to somewhere, the existence of Indigeneity in one's ancestral line is not the same as the lived experience of Indigeneity in this lifetime. Many of us with mixed ancestry need to spend time reflecting on this distinction. To claim Indigeneity is to claim the experiences of Indigenous peoples. While there is value and importance to being in solidarity, it is harmful to take on an identity that isn't yours.

For example, I have Indigenous Mexican blood on my father's side and mixed European ancestry on my mother's side. Like many of us, I live with feet in multiple worlds and have inherited both the trauma of assimilation and the moral injury of colonization. I was raised in the suburbs of Portland, Oregon, cut off from connection with my father's side of the family. As a white-passing Mexican person living in Oregon, I was raised with no direct connection to the struggle of the Indigenous people of Mexico, including my grandparents and their families. It is possible that my ancestors had connections to both peyote and psilocybin medicine practices.

Part of my work in this lifetime is to mend the broken connections and learn about the cultural practices and lifeways we were separated from. But I must do this repair work while acknowledging my privilege as a white-passing person and take care not to take up space occupying the identity of an Indigenous person or appropriating practices or customs that are not mine to hold. Indigeneity is not an identity you can put on and take off; it is a lifeway and belonging to a people. It is not about who you claim; it is about who claims you. It is about language, land, culture, custom, dance, community, and relationship.

In the psychedelic field, there is an overidentification with Indigeneity that can be harmful to First Nations peoples from around the world. This field has a complicated history with its relationship to Indigenous leadership. What I have witnessed in just a few years has ranged from extractive, exploitative, and performative to sincere and reparative.

It's not uncommon for non-Indigenous individuals who feel strong connections to medicine work to focus on their perceived entitlements: to participate in sacred customs such as cacao ceremonies, serve sacred medicines, share songs, live in holy places, or wear traditional attire. As a result, key reflections are missed and can crowd out deeper considerations that deserve our collective energy. Rather than centering our own intentions, feelings of connection, or entitlement to certain practices, members of the psychedelic field can instead reflect on how we find ourselves in the struggle for Indigenous sovereignty and thriving, both locally and in communities around the world who steward the medicines we love.

Consider how you can be of service to uplift Indigenous-led efforts for land justice, climate justice, sovereignty, and self-determination. These are life-and-death struggles playing out today that impact all of us. Get in relationship with water and land protectors in your area. Educate yourself about the struggles in the Amazon. Engage with groups working to conserve sacred medicines. Participation is a part of reciprocity.

As psychedelic practice grows more widespread, it's important that we give extra attention to these colonial dynamics within ourselves and our communities, and compassionately hold ourselves accountable. Start within.

In Conversation with Miriam Volat

One group working to change the colonial present is the Indigenous Peyote Conservation Initiative (IPCI), which is working to secure a future for Indigenous access to and participation in sacred plant medicine and pilgrimage. The IPCI conservation effort exists to sustain the spiritual practices of Indigenous peoples for generations to come, "promoting health, well-being, and Native cultural revitalization through sovereignty and sustainability of the Sacred Peyote plant and the lands on which it grows."[33] Their core strategy for confronting the peyote crisis consists of community engagement, promoting regrowth, replanting, changing policy, and land owner incentivization. IPCI currently has campsites and a bathhouse on the conservation lands that all Native Americans can use as a place of sacred pilgrimage to the peyote gardens.

The work being done by IPCI is fundamentally tied to Indigenous sovereignty and cultural revitalization. Fighting back against complex effects of colonization and the racist drug war, IPCI is working to secure a future for Indigenous spiritual practice and culture against economic, political, and racial boundaries. The IPCI is asserting Indigenous legal sovereignty by moving forward with spiritual and ecological supply of their medicine. The group is asserting Indigenous cultural sovereignty by providing access to pilgrimage and changing the colonial present, and asserting ecological sovereignty by taking back stewardship of the land in order to ensure that their sacrament can sustain itself.

There are two important ways Indigenous leaders have called on the psychedelic field to help ensure future Indigenous access to sacred peyote medicine: first, leave it out of decriminalization efforts, and second, donate directly to Indigenous-led conservation and stewardship efforts. On a larger level, we must urge our government to loosen economic and legal restrictions on the peyote market in order to encourage cultivation and growth in the number of distributors and pickers to improve restoration of the species and access for Indigenous peyote users. When it comes to this medicine in particular, the most important factors are respect for the plant as a living being, the land on which it grows, and the traditions and communities most impacted by its decline. It is critical to take action in order to preserve the sanctity and continuity of this rich and transformative healing tradition.

Miriam is codirector of the RiverStyx Foundation and director of the Indigenous Medicine Conservation Fund. She is also executive director of IPCI. Miriam works as a facilitator, educator, and community organizer to increase broad-based community and ecological resilience and decolonize philanthropy. Her work focuses on the intersection of biological and sociocultural diversity. She has never stopped exploring nutrient cycles and soil ecology, the emphasis of her MS work in the UC Davis Vegetable Crops Department. She also has degrees in political science and environmental studies.

Her life's work at RiverStyx includes supporting efforts that allow issues stigmatized by society to be worked with in a way that brings healing. This includes supporting radical composting efforts as well as Indigenous medicine, land, and cultural conservation. RiverStyx is committed to supporting a healthful integration of powerful medicines into society in a way that does no harm. As a mom, she is fortunate her daughter, Cora, also supports her work and participates passionately in her many adventures.

RM: *How did you come into working within or adjacent to the psychedelic field?*

MV: Well, my background is in ecology, and particularly soils. I decided to study soils, partly because I was really interested in contemporary philosophy around how humans interact with their home as a source of sustenance. I'm also somebody who grew up without going to school until I was a teenager, and most of my time was spent outside—which I consider to be one of the really lucky parts of my life. So I was really brought up by the environment, the ecosystem that I lived in.

I arrived at wanting to study philosophy around the age of twelve or thirteen, partly because of the shock of discovering that what a lot of humans were doing was really destructive to their homes. This was deeply shocking. From that, I decided to focus on food systems. At that time, I also had a fascination with how soils work and microbiology. I wanted to learn about the difference between a living soil and a dead soil. It was an intellectual interest that I had (and I just love working in the dirt!). So I had the good fortune of getting to study soils on a hundred-year project at UC Davis, and ended up getting my degree in nutrient cycling and agroecosystems.

Another personal thread for me was that I love to work with water and my personal kind of sacred boundaries were around water. Witnessing water pollution was where my initial shock as a child came from about what humans were doing to our environment. So my particular technical thread in agriculture was focused on preventing nonpoint source pollution to water systems from agroecosystems. I started working on climate action plans for particular agriculture industries. And so we'd gather farm labor groups, environmental groups, agencies, large farmers, small farmers, activists. We'd get everybody together and do pre-policy work.

I've taught small farming, but from more of a cultural perspective, looking at whole systems. Asking, how do we create culture where people feed and clothe and house themselves in a way that doesn't harm their home?

Working on water, something that is so core sacred, has held a lot of parallels to working on medicines. Because, how do you work in a "multi-stakeholder," or diverse multicultural setting with lots of different agendas, lots of complexity, and money issues bumping into cultural issues? How do you work with something that's really, really sacred, in a format that is decidedly not sacred—meaning out in the public, all over the place?

For me, there's some way that working on psychedelics, working on plant medicines, supporting Indigenous people in their way of life being intact in the new world that's emerging . . . for me personally, it is still my water work. That remains my core commitment.

Where and from whom are we learning how to not harm our home and our waters? Well, it is the Indigenous communities still connected to the land that help create this knowledge base we need.

I was actually running a compost toilet research project. For a while I was trying to get composting toilets to be legal in California, for people to not shit in water. And I've always been really interested in the psychological impact for people to actually be part of a cycle. So when you go to the bathroom in a bucket, and then you add your carbon, and then take the steps to take care of it, and it becomes soil, there's something different that happens to your understanding of the cycles that you're in. Where your food comes from and where it goes.

Believe it or not, that's how I got into working in the psychedelic space. I didn't know before that people were working with psychedelics on things like end-of-life care. The cancer anxiety trials that happened fourteen years ago at Johns Hopkins, where basically what was happening is that people were using psilocybin. And of course I love fungi, because if you're a soil scientist, you know that they are super, super-cool! And they were working with mushrooms (or at least part of the mushrooms) to help people adjust their experience of what death is. People who are comfortable with natural cycles tend to have a different relationship to death.

So I was super-lit up! And then Cody, my codirector at RiverStyx said, "Well, you've done all this multi-stakeholder facilitation on water. Can I support you to come to Laredo and meet with the NCNAC [National Council of Native American Churches]?" So I went through a whole process of planning for these meetings. And it was just hilarious, because I would call these leaders and ask them, "What are your intended outcomes for the meeting?" And they would be like, "Intended outcomes?" Having lived in some of those communities before, I knew I needed to adjust my approach.

They decided to form a conservation organization and asked me to be the interim director, until they had an Indigenous person to run it. And that's how I came into the medicine space.

And with the peyote work, it's so nuanced. It's a place where a lot of different tribes can come together and have incredible success with what a lot of the elders have said is the only thing left that hasn't been taken away from them. I see it as incredibly important for the US psychedelic community. *Because if the psychedelic community actually conducts themselves in a way that is respectful to the change process that's happening in Indigenous communities, and they don't jump the gun, and they don't do the usual colonial interference, it will actually bring more healing than any one psychedelic trip could ever have— it would be a cultural healing in this country.*

RM: *Something I see missing from a lot of the psychedelic field is a deep connection to actual, real-world culture, belonging, sense of place, and a sense of groundedness in the land as our home. It feels sort of fringe and dismissed in this field sometimes, talking about real-world healing, which means healing our history, healing our relationship to the living world that we're a part of.*

MV: As a movement, we're in this stage where the emphasis is on personal healing. And the assumption that, "Of course that's what we're doing" is actually super-fascinating. And I think it's worth deconstructing a bit, because you could actually look at it as completely the other way around.

Like . . . why all the emphasis on personal healing when you aren't even going to have clean water? I hear this a lot in the psychedelic movement. I'm not saying it's wrong, but the idea that if you haven't done your work, then you can't be doing other things. I just think it's worth questioning the order of priorities, or the intent that we have. Is there an order to things on personal versus collective healing? Do they happen at the same time? You know, how do you attend to both?

I think one of the reasons the peyote work has been so fraught the past few years is because there is this really profound potential community healing aspect to it. And it is a different order of priorities than most of the psychedelic movement.

RM: *It makes me think of when you have a wound needing to be cleaned out, that's been allowed to fester. And because of that, cleaning it out is so painful and gruesome. And in the same way, the bigger the potential reparative impact and the greater the stakes, the greater a reaction or resistance when these things try to come into the world. I also find that really energizing too; as ugly as it can be, it's that edge of potential for us to tell a new story.*

MV: That brings up another thing I think is so important at this moment, which is respect. There are many ways that word is so important. My experience is that if you lean into any of these medicines and our relationship with them, the layers of healing that you're gonna get into are pretty profound.

I think it's really okay for us to err on the side of caution. Just as in food systems, to utilize the precautionary principle. Not to avoid being brave and move toward things, but to move with our eyes and ears open, to be checking things out and knowing you might need to course-correct. We have to respect these medicines. The human mind and our connection with the rest of the chemistry of the planet is really incredible. So having a lot of respect. Play and fun aren't necessarily counter to that, but I think it's okay to be a little slow and careful.

And then if we slow down, we can see that there are many more voices about how nature works. There are still intact threads of knowledge about how to actually harmonize and integrate with nature. Things we might not have learned as a kid, depending on how we were raised. What if I listen? It takes time to temper all that excitement. Then this beautiful thing happens when we start to relax into the moment and learn how to corral that energy. That is the pacing and the rhythm of respect. Jumping the gun can get us into places where you're out of respect with the power of these medicines, out of sync with our own process of getting the most healing from them, healing having the broadest definition and not just being about you feeling better in the world.

RM: *When you say the broadest definition of healing, what does that mean for you? What comes to mind when you imagine what that could be?*

MV: For me, I see the broadest definition of healing in this lifetime to mean harmony as physical beings with our home, the earth. I think we all hold different pieces of that; it's a very big thing. There are our human relationships or animal relationships. If I had a wish for everybody's healing, it would be for people to be tending their connection to the earth, and their place on it. It's just that simple. I guess it's not that complicated.

We have to have direct experience. Sometimes the experience can just be subtle and one time and it'll create a cascade of changes. But it's one of the reasons why I spent a lot of time doing experiential outdoor education, was trying to understand what gives somebody an experience of connectivity that they can replicate, recognize, and build on and see little glimpses of and then fan it along. I don't think it takes much. I think that's one of the things some of these medicines can do, is provide people with an experience of feeling connected or feeling held, and then that has incredible ripple effects. One of the things I love about some of the psychedelics is that it can break down that dichotomy. To illuminate that those things aren't mutually exclusive.

That's one of the reasons why I'm so deeply committed to the Indigenous work and why we started the Indigenous Medicine Conservation (IMC) Fund. We've talked about climate change, but as we all know, that's just a small part of it. We're losing massive amounts of biodiversity. We're in the midst of the sixth great extinction. And I've been learning more about how to speak about this in the psychedelic space.

From a global perspective, we can't lose any more cultures, especially cultures that actually have the knowledge of their own places that make it so that humans aren't separate from their ecosystem. So there is an urgency not to lose any more places from a biodiversity and cultural diversity perspective. We can't afford to lose any more places, people, communities, or cultures that have knowledge about how to live in a way that honors that we're not separate. Part of what I think the psychedelic experience can do is help us recognize that there are things beyond us that are more important. Like biodiversity. And cultural diversity is directly tied to biodiversity, because 80 percent of the land that holds the most biodiversity is tended or supposed to be tended by cultural peoples who still have some of their cultural ways intact. This is not a little deal.

Conclusion

When we pause to really sit with the history of what has occurred, both in our lifetime and lifetimes past, it feels almost trite to promote reciprocity. It is not enough. It is offering a token of appreciation in the face of immeasurable pain, suffering, and injustice. So much more is needed. Reciprocity is harm-reduction on a community level—a way of being present with the weight of all that has occurred and finding what is within your power to contribute toward less harm, to contribute toward healing.

Reciprocity will not be perfect—relationships are not perfect. And it is not a remedy to repair the harms that have occurred. Not all reciprocity is visible. While practical, sincere offerings such as meaningful gifts, financial resources, time, labor, prayer, support, and solidarity are all forms of reciprocity, so is the inner-work we do in private: the work of unlearning colonial beliefs and ways of thinking and acting. Taking the time to examine where the Natural Colonial Gaze shows up in each of our lives and taking steps to be different. These are also forms of reciprocity. They are an acknowledgment of the people who have carried this medicine, to our great benefit today. We can show our gratitude to the medicines themselves by getting to know them—who they grew up with, where they come from, and who they call family. Reciprocity begets humility and humility begets reciprocity. And the sense of groundedness, clarity, and belonging that come from right relationship are the medicine our world needs.

Ultimately, as we reseed this essential practice or reciprocity into our habits and culture, it can evolve from a series of intentional actions into a whole way of being. Without reciprocity there is no such thing as whole medicine.

CHAPTER 13

Hope

In the first year I spent building Alma Institute, I had to continuously reckon with a tangled mess of hopefulness, frustration, and despair. We were two years into the pandemic and confronting not only the challenges of helping create a regulated psilocybin access program for which we have no real-world reference points; we were also contending with being a brand new nonprofit in a difficult philanthropic landscape during a financial downturn.

I remember many nights lying awake and wondering if we were going to make it. So many of us had poured our hearts, energy, health, spirits, and finances into bringing Alma into the world. I want to recognize my mentor, friend, and Alma's lead curriculum designer, Diana Quinn, ND, who shouldered so much of the labor of birthing this program and without whom it simply would not exist.

What we wanted to do seemed impossible. With every success, we encountered another roadblock: regulatory hurdles, health challenges, family shifts, financial scarcity, public pressure to move faster, and the forces of misogyny and white supremacy that couldn't seem to comprehend a group of ambitious women of color actually succeeding at what they'd set out to do: create a psychedelic training program and service center by and for marginalized communities and our allies.

During this time, we couldn't afford not to engage with hope. There were plenty of days when hope was the only thing keeping our team intact and preventing me from calling the whole thing off. On my most precarious days, I would call in sick. I would sit at my altar and cry or wander the neighborhood for hours, waiting for the spark of inspiration to return, for some sign that we were still on the path. When I got quiet enough, I could usually find it. When I couldn't, I called on my inner circle or mentors to drum it up for me.

Somehow, we fumbled through for sixteen months and came into our launch season joyful and a little worse for wear. It cost us more than we had prepared for (in every sense), and many of us on the team had long healing roads ahead, a process of unwinding the tensions in our hearts, spirits, and bodies of holding such precious medicine under the crushing forces of colonial capitalist culture. I'm still in awe of the fact that we made it this far; it wasn't guaranteed.

The only answer I have is that the medicines got under our skin. They showed us something we couldn't unsee, a mirage of possibility that was so heart-achingly beautiful and real that it was worth the risk: a future where the medicines that had been weaponized could return to being allies for healing. A new-yet-ancient era where communities would determine the shape of that healing for themselves, led by their hearts and supported by inner-work, accountability, and the distribution of power. A season of reconciliation, repair, and possibility. They asked us to show up for our own healing over and over so we could show up for our shared purpose with one another.

The medicines had inoculated us with hope. And in my experience, it's a fuel that burns a lot cleaner than anger.

The Tenacity of Hope

Hope doesn't preclude feeling sadness or frustration or anger or any other emotion that makes total sense. Hope isn't an emotion, you know? Hope is not optimism. Hope is a discipline . . . we have to practice it every single day.[1]

—MARIAME KABA

It's hard to know how to bring this book to a close. We have covered a whole lot of ground together. Thank you for sticking around this long and for doing the hard work to stay present through such weighty material. I hope that what we've offered up in these pages can help nudge us toward the psychedelic field and communities our hearts believe are possible.

Before we part ways, I want to share some reflections on one final element of practice: Hope.

The longer I work in this space, the heavier the work feels. Not just the weight of all that needs to be healed and transformed in the world, but also the weight of responsibility on those of us who are in the psychedelic field to help shape it in a good way. The sense of distrust, fear, regret, uncertainty, and futility can all weigh heavily and sometimes be immobilizing.

And yet, as has been demonstrated in so many important movements throughout history, in both the natural world and the narrative arc of human life, hope is a tenacious force as strong as life. It's in our bones. I believe that hope is more than an emotion or a superpower that descends on some of us and not on others; it's not just an emotion we feel when the clouds part or good news comes our way. In a deep way, hope is also a practice, and it relies on a web of relationships to hold it.

For me, hope requires that I first come back to center and find my heart. It insists that I get quiet. The medicines can help us do this too. When I set down all the burdens I am carrying and release the weight of the world's suffering, I can access a flicker of possibility deep in my rib cage that never seems to go out. Perhaps it is tied up with optimism. It's also tied up with presence; it involves accessing "okayness" wherever I can find it—in my body or my surroundings—as a reminder that, in fact, this is not the end of the world. Sometimes I need other people to remind me of this because I'm too weary to see it myself.

That flicker suggests that, in spite of all the ugliness and uncertainty, there is something worth carrying on toward. Hope feels like looking out at a clear-cut forest and remembering that the soil is still teeming with life and the generative forces of regrowth.

Hope can also be a bit elusive. In my experience, hope tends to emerge when it's no longer something that would be nice to have, it's something absolutely necessary in order to carry on. It's the matchbook I go digging for in my closet when the power goes out. In other words, I don't feel a lot of hope when I'm lukewarm or ambivalent about situations. I feel hope (or its absence) most palpably when the stakes are high and I'm already in a freefall toward despair. And it's usually given to me by someone I love who is close enough to notice me unraveling.

Hope on its own is vulnerable to being reduced to a sentiment of positive outlook. The hope we are talking about is more than that. It is the audacious dreaming that generates action.

Holding Hope

The role of community in stoking the flames of hope cannot be overstated. Our shared visions are more than the sum of their parts; when we weave them together, we strengthen a fabric of our commitment, as well as belief in the possibility and beauty of what we hope to achieve.

Hope is not an individual endeavor. Ideally, it's something we take turns tending, as the central fire in the village. We can't rely on just a few of us to hold it for everyone. Check on those you turn to for navigation through hopeless times. Healthy movements need webs of support so that even the most prominent leaders can have space to fall apart and be fully human. This softness in itself is revolutionary.

PERSONAL

We each hold a deeply personal relationship to our own hopes and dreams. These may be visions for who we want to become and the lives we want to shape for ourselves and those we love. We might come to the medicines out of the hope that we can heal something specific ailing us, or we might simply be carried forward by the belief that we are not yet complete; that there is still time for becoming.

PSYCHEDELIC

If you've read this far, I imagine we are aligned in our hope of creating a psychedelic field reflective of humane values. The best way I have found to deal with concerns about corporate foolishness is to put our attention into creating alternatives. Let's render problematic structures obsolete. Hope doesn't come from hand-wringing and writing spicy comments on Instagram about patents and retreat prices. In my experience, hope is fed by meaningful action in the direction we want to move.

Releasing perfectionism also creates more elasticity and room for hope, instead of viewing each policy or new development in our field from a binary mindset of "it's the ideal or it's evil." Not everyone is on board with the slow crawl of incrementalism. We need the idealists to help steer us in the direction of best-case scenarios. However, those who hold this role are prone to becoming jaded and burnt out. That's because transformation doesn't often happen in the realm of best-case scenarios. It happens in iterations. It often looks more like: two steps forward, one step back, learn, unlearn, reconsider, evolve, make shifts, and repeat. There is no room for these important phases in all-or-nothing thinking.

Change is unfolding all around us constantly. With this awareness, we can aspire to stay present, relax our field of vision, and remain engaged in the work even when things go the opposite of how we believe they should. Nothing is fixed in place. Even missteps are part of a larger unfolding and can provide critical insights to guide us. Each milestone is a chance to rest, reflect, gather collective wisdom, and nurture our hope before continuing on.

I believe if enough of us commit to our inner-work and embrace tenacious hope as a practice, we will inevitably create the psychedelic future we are after: a thriving, diverse ecosystem marked by justice, community healing, access, safety, resilience, and integrity. For this to happen, we need to remain at the table and keep bridges intact (in spite of imperfect settings), long enough to influence the way things are done.

COLLECTIVE

We already have what we need to thrive on this generous planet. We humans are getting in our own way. When we zoom out and reflect on the grander arc of history, we can see the distinct crises of our times, which call for immediate, planet-wide, societal harm-reduction. Our first priority is to stop the bleeding. But we also hold the potential for much more beyond just mitigating disaster. Imagine a time on the horizon when our focus shifts to thriving rather than simply healing. It's a bold dream, but one shared among many.

Often, social change takes generations. Part of our ability to hold onto hope comes from acceptance that we are part of a much slower, larger unfolding. Our imaginations paint a picture for us of the story our children and their children could tell. Even if the image is blurry or humble, it's the worthy story of how we carried the torch of change in our lifetimes. The moment of history is marked, in addition to so many interlocking injustices, by a fifty-year drug war that suppressed culture, community, justice, and life. By a mass extinction beyond any scale in human history. By an era of extreme imbalances in every system we rely upon to sustain life. This could be the pressure under which hope bloomed and flipped the script.

Hope insists that the story isn't over. With all the talk in recent years about the end of the world, the apocalypse, and global collapse, these deflating narratives indulge our desire to surrender to despair. We can scratch the itch for a moment, but doing so asks us to disregard the unencumbered forces of life that are very much still here with us.

HOPE AS A CLEAN-BURNING FUEL

In a 2021 interview with *Intercepted,* healing justice leader Mariame Kaba said:

> And that became a mantra for me when I would feel unmoored. Or when I would feel overwhelmed by what was going on in the world, I would just say to myself: "Hope is a discipline." It's less about "how you feel," and more about the practice of making a decision every day, that you're still gonna put one foot in front of the other, that you're still going to get up in the morning. And you're still going to struggle, that was what I took away from it.

> It's work to be hopeful. It's not like a fuzzy feeling. You have to actually put in energy, time, and you have to be clear-eyed, and you have to hold fast to having a vision. It's a hard thing to maintain. But it matters to have it, to believe that it's possible to change the world. You know, that we don't live in a predetermined, predestined world where like nothing we do has an impact. No, no, that's not true! Change is, in fact, constant, right? Octavia Butler teaches us. We're constantly changing. We're constantly transforming. It doesn't mean that it's necessarily good or bad. It just is. That's always the case. And so, because that's true, we have an opportunity at every moment to push in a direction that we think is actually a direction towards more justice.[2]

Hope enables the imagination exercises required to dream forward a future we can love. It fuels the visions of what is possible. Sometimes it means setting aside all the valid reasons we have to *not* be optimistic, not trust, and not try. To be visionary is to water the seeds of hope, and to embrace both the thrill of dreaming and the tenderness of vulnerability.

When leveraged as fuel for our collective liberation, hope is a tenacious force. It's the refusal to give in to despair or to let dominant systems win out. What a fierce, beautiful thing! I believe we can go further by relating to hope not only as a discipline, but also as an outcome of celebratory practices.

WONDER AND CELEBRATION

Hope is something that can multiply upon itself once it is set in motion. But from a vacuous place where so many communities find themselves, pointing to hope can be akin to telling people to "cheer up." Hope can be hard to access when there is no visible proof that change is possible. Cynicism makes sense; it's a sound trauma response.

While hope is a practice and something we cultivate over time, it doesn't seem fruitful to tell people hope is another thing they need to work on. Life is about more than hard work and reckoning with pain; when the wounds get cleared out, we also get to fill the empty space with good things. These cycles of breaking down and building back up are innate to us as living beings.

Hope thrives in a positive feedback loop. We need to feel it in our bodies and have access points for the lives we are individually and collectively healing into. So the question is, how might we access hope in a roundabout way? *What are the experiences that can facilitate hope?*

In order to carry on with powerful transformative work, we need opportunities to soften and take the edge off. It doesn't have to be earned. I'm curious about what can happen when we find ways to collectively shield ourselves from the onslaughts of dominant culture, even if just for a moment, and immerse ourselves in the experiences that foster joy and belonging. What happens when we make this a habit? We know that resistance is critical. But we also need to know, not only in our minds but in our bodies and hearts, *how our liberation is also contained in pleasure,* through the vehicles of rest, celebration, wonder, awe, connection, laughter, stillness, and all the magical things taken by systems of domination. *This is why the celebratory and sensual spaces we create for ourselves are never frivolous. They're medicine.* Psychedelics can enhance these spaces, but they're not at all required.

What these spaces look like is up to us; there are infinite possibilities and many people in our communities are already living into them. A few patterns emerge: gathering, feasting, music, dance, and personal connection are our human heritage. Fill in whatever feels important for you. I'd like to see these elements more woven into our healing spaces, to dissolve the distinctions between healing and living.

In the outro of her gorgeous book *Pleasure Activism,* author and healing justice practitioner adrienne maree brown writes:

> True pleasure—joy, happiness and satisfaction—has been the force that helps us move beyond the constant struggle, that helps us live and generate futures beyond this dystopic present, futures worthy of our miraculous lives.

> Pleasure—embodied, connected pleasure—is one of the ways we know when we are free. That we are always free. That we always have the power to cocreate the world. Pleasure helps us move through the times that are unfair, through grief and loneliness, through the terror of genocide, or days when the demands are just overwhelming. Pleasure heals the places where our hearts and spirits get wounded. Pleasure reminds us that even in the dark, we are alive. Pleasure is a medicine for the suffering that is absolutely promised in life.[3]

Ceremony is intrinsic to life.
Life is not separate from suffering.
Suffering is entangled with pleasure.
Pleasure is intertwined with ceremony.

And on and on we go; living with pleasure is a generative cycle. We're not just talking about integration; we're talking about seeding a culture of hope through daily actions that foreshadow the lives we're dreaming into. What a gift to ourselves, our ancestors, and our descendants.

In Conversation with Bill Brennan

I was relaxing in an entheogenic garden in Oakland, California, thumbing through a copy of Chacruna Institute's anthology, *Psychedelic Justice,* when I came across an essay that nearly popped off the page: "The Revolution Will Not Be Psychologized: Psychedelics' Potential for Systemic Change," by Bill Brennan.[4]

"Exactly!" I said out loud to no one. This was my first introduction to Bill's work, and because of this alignment in paradigms, I was glad to speak with him for this book. In this conversation we spoke about the limitations of individual mental healthcare, the implications of dosing for productivity, and the potential for psychedelics to help us heal root causes of systemic injustice . . . if we hold those efforts together as communities.

Bill Brennan, PhD, is a psychologist in New York City. He is a codeveloper of the EMBARK approach to psychedelic-assisted therapy and has served as core faculty and clinical supervisor for psychedelic clinical trials that have used EMBARK. He works as a consultant for several psychedelic treatment development companies where he has coauthored several treatment manuals. He is a member of the legislative committee of the New York Psilocybin Action Committee, a group that works toward the decriminalization of psilocybin and other psychedelics. His interests are at the intersection of psychedelics and liberatory approaches that contribute to systemic change.

RM: *In your article for Chacruna you said, "Consider how many of our lethal epidemics, depression, suicide, addiction, gun violence, have systemic causes, they get lost in our public conversations about increasing access to the panacea of mental health services. For these and many other issues, we have hamstrung our imagination for broader change by locating the root of suffering within the individual."*

What kinds of possibilities do you think we might be missing out on by not engaging with our imaginations, and by not looking beyond the current Band-Aids that we have?

BB: I'd be wary of any answer that I come up with personally, because I'm just one person. These answers really have to be something that comes out of a collective. That being said, there's one idea that I put forth in the article from [Ignacio] Martin-Baró about turning people toward confronting the sources of their suffering, instead of just aiming to alleviate their suffering, in psychotherapy. We could call this a kind of consciousness raising. That's something that we could focus work into our approaches to psychotherapy. So, it feels like one of the closer possibilities.

There are different ways to define "individualism." We could say that our preoccupation with our own healing and happiness without considering the broader context is a kind of "passive" individualism. There's also a more "active" individualism, which is a more competitive attitude of, "Screw everybody else; I'm gonna do my best to take what I can take and to succeed where I can." And I think that's why many of us in the world of psychedelics look so askance at individualistic psychedelic culture, because it is very much about gaining that competitive advantage and it veers into a more active form of individualism.

RM: *To get ahead or to advance implies getting ahead of others or climbing on others or winning out. People might not see it that way; they might just be thinking, I want success. In your view, can individual therapy actually reinforce the status quo?*

BB: At its core, it reframes collective problems in individual terms. *If you were to keep pulling on the threads coming off of the problems people bring to therapy,*

you'd eventually see the ways in which structural or systemic factors are contrib-
uting to or even causing many of them. Psychotherapy can focus us away from
that fact and turn our focus onto individual-level solutions as a place to put our
energies. And what we see happening now, especially among younger generations, is a real emphasis on "mental health" as a sort of solution to everything.

This reframing happens at the individual level in regard to how we think
about our own suffering. It also impacts how we think about the suffering of
other people that we're close to and connected to. And then, at the broader
level, if we recognize that there's a problem, something like gun violence
or suicidality, our knee-jerk reaction is to ask, "What can we do to increase
access to mental healthcare?" *It has given us an easy answer to a lot of questions
that shouldn't and don't have easy answers.*

On one hand, we still haven't figured out how to give access to basic
mental healthcare to everyone who could benefit from it. So, it's still a challenge. But, on the other hand, it has become "easy" in the sense that it is a
widely known practice with clearly defined lines around it. We know what
it looks like to do psychotherapy, we know what it looks like to open mental
health clinics, and we know the mechanisms for increasing or decreasing
funding for mental health. There is already a set of parameters and a set of
actors that are operating around it.

Whereas the solutions that might benefit us most are those that don't
have clear lines pointing to them. So mental health services give us something to point to when we don't know where else to point.

In psychotherapy there's been this decades-long campaign against the
stigma of mental health challenges, and the stigma of seeking and receiving
psychotherapy. That's been a beautiful, necessary battle. And it's been won
to a large extent. But like so many other things that have won that battle of
public acceptance, it was immediately subsumed by the spectacle. It's been
appropriated and incorporated into the larger set of strategies that can actually keep us from effecting any kind of real change.

RM: *Like you spoke about earlier, this practice of turning awareness into meaningful action could be applied to confronting so many current challenges: food
systems, healthcare, racial oppression, climate justice. Why do you think we're
not engaging with psychedelics to help us turn our attention toward and address
these more widespread challenges?*

BB: It should certainly be more a part of the conversation. I think my concern, specifically in the realm of psychedelics, is that there is, as we know, a suggestibility-
enhancing effect of psychedelics. I think it's such a tricky thing, because I want

to say something like: "We could use psychedelics to build solidarity in a group of people who are trying to organize a union in their workplace" or something like that. But the counterpoint is that you could just as easily use psychedelics to indoctrinate people into oppressive belief systems. It could be fascist solidarity, or it could be liberationist solidarity. These are the questions we have to grapple with when we talk about using psychedelics for the sake of the collective.

In Conversation with Ismail Ali

For my last interview, I spoke with a dear friend and trusted colleague, Ismail Lourido Ali. In addition to being one of the more recognized leaders in psyche-delic policy reform, Ismail—whose friends call him Izzy—has been a thought partner and confidant, and has strongly influenced my orientation to this work. He has built bridges between the worlds of psychedelics and drug policy, and has managed to stay actively engaged in the work for many years, in spite of the many challenges presented by this nascent field.

Ismail has utilized psychedelics and other drugs and substances in celebratory, social, and spiritual contexts for more than half his life. He began actively partici-pating in the drug policy reform movement ten years ago, and today is the director of policy and advocacy at the Multidisciplinary Association of Psychedelic Studies (MAPS). Ismail also currently serves on the board of directors for Alchemy Com-munity Therapy Center (formerly Sage Institute) in California's Bay Area and is a cofounder and current board member of the Psychedelic Bar Association. Ismail advises, is formally affiliated with, or has served in leadership roles for other orga-nizations in the drug policy reform ecosystem, including Students for Sensible Drug Policy, Chacruna Institute, and the Ayahuasca Defense Fund, all in service to envi-sioning and designing a safe and compassionate post-prohibition world.

RM: *At the Women's Visionary Congress in 2019, you began with an imagination exercise. You asked the audience to imagine a world that is just. I'd love to hear where that came from, or why it felt important for you to start with that exercise before you gave your talk.*

IA: I can't take credit for the exercise. I heard it somewhere else sometime in the month or two before that event. And I remember thinking, "This is a really beautiful exercise that we should practice as a field." The question put out to the group was: "What would it be like if the world was just?" And more spe-cifically, "What would *you* be doing if the world was just?"

I have a friend and mentor whom I met when I was in law school. They were the first person to tell me that they believed that their responsibility was to work themselves out of a job. And I asked, "What does that mean?" And they said, "Well, I work in immigration reform. I would like to work toward a paradigm in which I don't have to defend people in this way anymore. I don't want us to always be in a place that starts from a premise of injustice that we then have to defend people against our own government." That really resonated with me.

Even considering the nonprofit industrial complex framework: so many of the pathways for social change that we're currently offered are still mitigated by wealth allocation. And frankly, they often require that you align with the needs and expectations of people with large amounts of wealth. Yes, there is actual concrete benefit from the system of philanthropy. But zooming out into the deeper purpose of social change work, the goal is not for me to perpetually have a job and be reliant on other people's generosity to fund that work.

The world that we're trying to create does not require us to constantly be in a fight for our collective basic survival. So that was really impactful for me as a law student, when I was exploring what it meant to work in the world of social change. *The point is not to work in social change; it's to work toward it, such that the work becomes obsolete.*

Allowing people to reflect on who they would be without having to solve the problems of the world is a good starting point for visionary thought. Because visioning thought doesn't require us to solve the problems of the world. It just requires us to tap into what we wish we could do, or who we really think we are at our core.

I find it helpful to reground that relationship to hope in our personal identity and path, rather than hinging hope on the imagined solutions to our problems. I think that people, myself included, sometimes get tied up in the solving of the problems. And that can be really disheartening. Anyone who's tried to solve any of these big social problems has been confronted with what feels like the futility of it. Because we're just individual people trying to figure out problems that are much bigger than us. But also because, even with collective thought and organizing, we don't have that many good answers to our problems right now.

We can imagine what the structure could be like. But when it comes to the practical, pragmatic, operational elements of enacting justice, I think that there's a gap between the visionary kind of hope and desires that many of us hold, and the capacity to articulate it in a realistic world. And that is heartbreaking. I think for a lot of activists, it's one of the things that leads to burnout and failure of groups to actualize their vision. Not because they don't have hope, are not smart or dedicated; they are. But because the problems we think we're trying to solve are so big and multilayered, that even if we pull one string in the knot, we're tightening other parts. So, how do we untangle it all at the same time?

RM: *We've been taught that hope is an emotion. It's something that we either have or we don't. I'm wondering if you have any thoughts around reframing hope more as a discipline or a practice.*

IA: This is something I've heard from many people. I think that Mariame Kaba in her Prison Culture work talks about cultivating hope as a practice. There are other movement leaders who have put hope and love in a similar category that's not just an emotional experience. It's a way of being that impacts our actions and our mindset.

This one is interesting for me. It's true for me in the sense that I do experience practicing hope as a discipline, including, and especially in the face of the constant demoralization that occurs in social change work. I'm a very optimistic person, and I still experience a lot of burnout from the negativity or the stagnation of some of the work that I'm involved in. And I'm saying that as someone who's in a field that actually does have wins.

But even as someone who believes in hope as a practice, I can sometimes find it difficult to put in the effort. Same with inspiration. I feel like people believe hope just will just show up when it needs to. And I've just known too many people that have died by suicide to believe that it's true. It doesn't reliably show up to clear the clouds of our emotional minds. It's actually something that we have to tend to. It's very precious and we have to protect it. Which is hard. It can be really exhausting for people who are already doing so much. They're already trying to maintain a relationship with oneself, loved ones, their community, organization, or movement. What do you mean, I also have to be in active relationship with this thing called hope? Like, why can't it just be there when I need it? I'm sympathetic to that.

And the discipline piece is interesting. I actually don't experience hope all of the time. And sometimes I don't even feel the capacity to want to cultivate it. But if I don't put in the energy and effort to cultivate it ahead of time, then it's not there when I need it. Hope has that sort of delayed gratification quality to it. I don't think it's something that just shows up when called on. But you really have to tend to it and strengthen it so it's available when it's needed.

And one thing that I think about a lot is also Mariame Kaba's quote: "Let this radicalize you rather than lead you to despair."[5] I really struggle with it. Despite being a perma-optimist, I am also (perhaps paradoxically) very quick to despair. People don't usually see that side of me, and I don't talk about that so openly. I'm trying to figure out how to talk about it in a way that doesn't reinforce the despair that everyone already has. There's a responsibility when people look to you. With public visibility, how do you hold hope in the times when you just don't have it? How do you say, "No, it's okay. It's gotta be okay," when you don't know whether it's going to be okay? Who the hell's gonna hold that voice?

RM: *How do we respond when a whole community looks to you and says, "Can you anchor us in vision so we can find the will to carry on?"*

IA: That's something people need to do. Because I think it's also humanizing. It's something I do struggle with, which is like, who has the responsibility? Whose responsibility is it to hold the hope?

I'm thinking about civil rights and social justice leaders throughout history. They must have had breakdowns. They must have fallen apart. But that is not really the narrative we get. It's not really the story of like the hero in the psyche or imagination of the movements. I guess that's the shadow side to this conversation: we have to figure out how to utilize hope without relying on the people we look up to and want to hang so much of our hope on.

RM: *I want to democratize and have everyone doing their part, and I recognize there are specific roles for a reason.*

IA: There's a tension. What does it mean to democratize those elements of leadership when people self-select into the roles that they want to play, or they're placed in them by their sociocultural conditioning and environment? There are many people who think they want to fulfill certain roles, but don't realize what they're committing to, and then they shirk their responsibilities when they're placed in them.

And I think there is this kind of glamorizing of certain kinds of leadership, including spiritual leadership. We have this sort of consumerification of the movement where being a self-proclaimed voice for something is equated with true leadership. And you get the accolades, you know, or the public perception. Today's internet culture doesn't help. But once push comes to shove, you're actually not ready or available to provide the kind of grounding and support that's really needed from that position. That can be really destabilizing for communities.

RM: *The weight of responsibility is real. I think it's really good to slow down and look at that; to spend that time fostering a culture where we take these roles more seriously and understand what it is we're signing up for and the sacrifices that* *are involved. We want to be sure we are actually dedicated and able to hold what we're being handed. Moments of, "If I had known what I was signing up for . . . I probably wouldn't have said yes. And yet I'm so glad I did." It's something I hear again, and again, from the folks who hold roles of responsibility or leadership in our movements.*

IA: Yeah, that also kind of goes back to your original question. Do any of us know what we're signing up for? Do we need to or want to know? Is it actually supportive for us to know? Maybe we don't need to look at the hugeness of what we're trying to accomplish. Maybe that's okay. To some extent, I sometimes feel like the movement is fueled by its own naive optimism. But we can reclaim that. *I'll take being called a naive optimist if it is what gives me the energy to wish for and work toward something different.*

CONCLUSION

What would it feel like if the world was just?

I wonder, how would we live, play, and organize if we knew a just world was on its way and that we were its cocreators?

Without ascribing to Western concepts of perfectionism and purity, we can let ourselves imagine an expansive world of psychedelic practice marked by dynamic balance, harmony, integration, and presence. Creating space for more: More life. More understanding. More attunement. More connection and compassion. Wholeness means that everything is present and accounted for. This means we find a way to welcome not only the love and light, but the whole spectrum of realities—thriving and suffering, from the highest peaks to unimaginable depths—without judgment. With whole medicine, we can expand within ourselves and within our communities. As we grow in our capacity, we create more space to bear witness to and handle not only the complexities of the human experience, but the unique and pressing crises of our times.

If we start from an ambition of global change, we will never begin or we will quit when we encounter obstacles. We will become casualties to the fantasies of idealism. We can't actually change the whole world; we are finite beings among billions. We are tiny specks within a very large, established system. We don't know how to comprehend, let alone influence, things at the global level.

However: If we can create space in our most intimate settings and spheres of influence to remember and embody the deeper truths that we want to drive the world, actual, immediate change becomes possible. Remember that the individual is collective and the collective is individual. So as we heal ourselves, we alter reality in some small way. We tug on the threads of reality in the directions of love and justice. When enough of us do, entire systems can actually start to shift. This is what social movements are. This is how we achieve widespread change: beginning within ourselves, organizing, and infusing deep medicine into our movements.

In order to do this, we need to slow down enough and create enough space from the grind to engage our imaginations together. We rebel against the forces of extractive capitalism and death culture by creating spaces to dream. Some days, this dream might only be a blurry image or a subtle impression. When that's true, we can slow down and tend to it. We can be with the unknowns. Other days, the truth of possibility is so expansive and lush that we offer a belly laugh up to the sky for ever having doubted. Either way, our collective imaginations can light the way.

Alongside uncertainty, we can take the first step, and resource ourselves enough to continue taking steps. We can find respite and indulge our despair and heartbreaks along the way. We can bear witness to the ways our action carries power, the same way droplets of water coalesce and eventually carve out riverbeds. We can rely on one another and our medicine allies to reignite our belief when we find ourselves bogged down by the weight of it all. We can invite the others. We can create culture and enjoy our lives along the way. Hope does not hinge on arriving at an imagined future; we can access it as we embody a just world right now.

Where We've Been

The Essential Elements of Practice laid out in this book are just a few of the makings of deeply healing psychedelic work. Whether you are a journeyer, a facilitator, a skeptic, or a longtime explorer, I hope these pages have inspired you, challenged you, and introduced you to some of the leading voices we can look to as the coming years unfold.

We have explored the importance of gaining awareness through inner-work and shadow exploration, the ways trauma and healing shape our ability to be present, and the importance of discernment in navigating the wild world of psychedelia.

We have grappled with the beauty and messiness of community, the container for so much learning around power, harm-reduction, and consent. We've looked at interpersonal dynamics and relationships as the spaces where we learn the most about ourselves and what needs healing.

We dove deep into the systemic matters of accountability, history, and reciprocity. We discovered how the drug war and Indigenous reciprocity are intricately linked, and heard from leading voices in the worlds of transformative justice and decolonization for truth-telling and guidance. We've tinkered with the fractal, micro-macro ways our psychedelic spaces reflect our society, and examined ways we can heal ourselves to heal the collective.

We learned that justice starts at home. We found that there are no shortcuts to reciprocity, healing, and relationship.

And here we are, with hope. I'll pose again: *What would it feel like if the world was just?*

I've purposefully left much of the conclusion and meaning-making up to you, dear reader. How has this exploration been for you? What did you resonate with, and where did you find resistance? What Essential Elements of Practice emerged for you that weren't discussed here? I invite you to spend some time with them.

What does whole medicine mean in your context? What is your part to play in it? I hope you will engage with your loved ones and communities and build upon the ideas explored here. Debate, grapple, push back, and lean in. Meditate on them during your journeys and see what emerges. Engage with your ceremonial practices; let these new and ancient ideas dance with your cells until they find a place to settle. Take what you need and leave the rest.

Remember, too, that healing doesn't always have to be a struggle. It can also be joyous, restful, and pleasurable. Find out what your path calls for in this season. Allow space for your medicine work to evolve, as it certainly will. Wherever you find yourself, see what it's like to savor the spaciousness you can find in this moment, this breath, this body, this life. Shrink the gap between life and ceremony until you find their confluence. Spend time there. Settle roots there. Make a home there.

Thank you for coming on this journey with me. Let's integrate.

ACKNOWLEDGMENTS

Thank you—

Gracias a los niños santos, con quienes he compartido los momentos más sagrados de mi vida.

To the ancestors, family members, elders, Indigenous lineage keepers, drug policy reformers, chemists, outlaws, activists, writers, educators, abolitionists, land tenders, harm-reductionists, researchers, and medicine people who have carried us to this moment. Without their courage, sacrifice, and generosity, the life I'm living would not exist.

To my friends and lifemates for the love, patience, direct experiences, and late-night conversations that shaped these pages: JJ Airuoyo, Ani Achugbue, Heidi Berg, Claudia Cuentas, Axcelle Campana, Krystal Meyer, Andi Bixel, Leandra Romero, Manuel Bonilla, Stacy Holtmann, Ismail Ali, Diana Quinn, and Fuat Keceli.

To my brilliant coauthor Juliette Mohr, whose dedication and integrity brought such depth to chapters 11 and 12, on History and Reciprocity. To the beloved, esteemed guests we'll meet within these pages; I am in awe of each of you. To my mentors, advisors, and trusted colleagues: Hanifa Nayo Washington, Britt Rollins, Matthew Ettinger, Haena Park, Sandor Iron Rope, Michelle Janikian, Inti García Flores, Leonard Pickard, Kerthy Fix, and Paul Kloss. Without you, I wouldn't last in the psychedelic field.

To Tim McKee and Jasmine Respess at North Atlantic Books, and my prereaders, Elizabeth Lazarre Kaplan, Annie Oak, and Juliette Mohr. You were there.

To my team at Alma Institute who transmute the ideas presented here into the embodied, gorgeous, messy work of collective healing every day. To all those who will train and journey with us in the years to come, and the heart-centered donors who take leaps of faith with us: you are bringing these dreams earthside.

To those who grow, harvest, make, and tend to the medicines with integrity. To the loved ones with whom I get to venture across sacred realms and come back more fully alive. To the medicines for all their kindness, tricks, simplicity, grandeur, and marvelous strangeness.

To my son Moses, who is the most effortlessly psychedelic and beautiful soul I know.

These people have taught me more about life, ceremony, community, interdimensional travel, and love in action than one could ever learn from books.

And to you, dear reader, for joining us on the whole medicine path.

NOTES

Preface

1 adrienne maree brown, *Emergent Strategy* (Chico, CA: AK Press, 2017), 2.

Chapter 3: Shadow

1 C. G. Jung, *Psychology and Religion: West and East (The Collected Works of C. G. Jung, Vol. 11)*, (Princeton, NJ: Princeton University Press, 1938), 131.
2 Kylea Taylor, *The Ethics of Caring: Finding Right Relationship to Clients* (Santa Cruz, CA: Hanford Mead, 1995), 161.
3 Hannah McLane and Emma Knighton, "Narcissism in the Psychedelic Ecosystem," Chacruna Institute talk, September 14, 2022, www.crowdcast.io/e/narcissism-in-the/register.

Chapter 4: Discernment

1 Women's Visionary Congress, "20 Safety Tips for Those Participating in Ceremonies That Use Psychoactive Substances," December 2014, https://visionarycongress.org/articles/wvc-articles/safety-tips-r3/.
2 Women's Visionary Congress, "What Elders Offer to Psychedelic Communities," February 2023, https://visionarycongress.org/articles/wvc-articles/what-elders-offer-to-psychedelic-communities-r9/.

Chapter 5: Community

1 Steven W. Cole, John P. Capitanio, Katie Chun, Jesusa M.G. Arevalo, Jeffrey Ma, and John T. Cacioppo, "Myeloid Differentiation Architecture of Leukocyte Transcriptome Dynamics in Perceived Social Isolation," *Proceedings of the National Academy of Sciences of the United States of America,* 112, no. 49 (November 23, 2015): 15142–7, https://pubmed.ncbi.nlm.nih.gov/26598672.

Chapter 6: Power

1 Cyndi Suarez, *The Power Manual* (British Columbia, Canada: New Society Publishers, 2018), 26.

Chapter 8: Harm-Reduction

1 Annie Oak, *The Manual of Psychedelic Support: A Practical Guide to Establishing and Facilitating Care Services at Music Festivals and Other Events,* 2nd ed. (San Jose, CA: Multidisciplinary Association for Psychedelic Studies [MAPS], 2017), https://maps.org/product/manual-of-psychedelic-support/. A must-read, industry-defining resource for event organizers, volunteers, and people who hold space.

2 Oak, *Manual of Psychedelic Support*, 20–24.
3 Justice Rivera and Shaan Lashun, *Towards Bodily Autonomy* (Self-published, 2023), vi.
4 D. Des Jarlais, "Harm Reduction in the USA: The Research Perspective and an Archive to David Purchase," *Harm Reduction Journal* 14, no. 51 (2017).
5 Rivera and Lashun, *Towards Bodily Autonomy*, 222.

Chapter 9: Consent

1 Sylvia Duckworth, "Wheel of Privilege and Power," www.rwuc.org/wp-content/uploads/2021/09/wheel.pdf. Adapted from Canadian Council for Refugees, https://ccrweb.ca/en/power-wheel-update.
2 Staci K. Haines, *The Politics of Trauma* (Berkeley, CA: North Atlantic Books, 2019), 11.
3 Robin Wall Kimmerer, "The 'Honorable Harvest': Lessons from an Indigenous Tradition of Giving Thanks," *Yes!*, November 26, 2015, www.yesmagazine.org/issue/good-health/2015/11/26/the-honorable-harvest-lessons-from-an-indigenous-tradition-of-giving-thanks.
4 Joshua White and Juliana Mulligan, "Questions to Discuss with a Prospective Psychedelic Facilitator," Fireside Project, June 30, 2022, https://firesideproject.medium.com/questions-to-discuss-with-a-prospective-psychedelic-facilitator-2e36bc932040.

Chapter 10: Accountability

1 Anti-Oppression Resource & Training Alliance (AORTA), https://AORTA.Coop.
2 Barnard Center for Research on Women, "What is Transformative Justice?" YouTube, March 11, 2020, www.youtube.com/watch?v=U-_BOFz5TXo.
3 *The Psychedologist*, "Consciousness—Positivity—Radio," thepsychedologist.com.
4 Leia Friedwoman, "How the Psychedelic Community Should Respond to Sexual Abuse," *Lucid News*, October 29, 2021, www.lucid.news/how-the-psychedelic-community-should-respond-to-sexual-abuse/.
5 Heather Plett, "How Do You Process Uncomfortable Information?" Centre for Holding Space, June 24, 2021, https://centreforholdingspace.com/how-do-you-process-uncomfortable-information-an-infographic/.
6 "Philly Stands Up Accountability Roadmap," https://everydayfeminism.com/wp-content/uploads/2018/11/phillystandsup-final.pdf.
7 Rebecca Martinez, "Accountability & Transformative Justice in the Psychedelic Space: A Roadmap for Change," June 9, 2021, *Psychedelics Today*, https://psychedelicstoday.com/2021/06/09/accountability-transformative-justice-in-the-psychedelic-space-a-roadmap-for-change/.
8 Mariame Kaba and Shira Hassan, *Fumbling Towards Repair* (Project NIA, 2019).
9 Joshua White and Juliana Mulligan, "Warning Signs When Selecting a Psychedelic Facilitator," Fireside Project, June 30, 2022, https://firesideproject.medium.com/warning-signs-when-selecting-a-psychedelic-facilitator-9b803b1b9fee; "Questions to Discuss with a Prospective Psychedelic Facilitator," Fireside Project, June 30, 2022, https://firesideproject.medium.com/questions-to-discuss-with-a-prospective-psychedelic-facilitator-2e36bc932040.
10 Juliana Mulligan, "Guide to Finding a Safe Ibogaine Clinic," 2019, Inner Vision Ibogaine, www.innervisionibogaine.com/findingaclinic.

Chapter 11: History

1 Juliette Mohr, "Psychedelic Extractivism: Distilling Indigeneity into Exchange Value," 2021, www.juliettemohr.digital/post/psychedelic-extractivism.

2 Ibram X. Kendi and Jason Reynolds, *Stamped from the Beginning* (New York: Bold Type Books, 2016).

3 Cedric Robinson, *Black Marxism: The Making of the Black Radical Tradition* (Chapel Hill: University of North Carolina Press, 1983), 2.

4 Robinson, *Black Marxism,* xii.

5 Tori Saneda and Michelle Field, *Cultural Anthropology: Legacy of Colonialism* (Bothell, WA: Cascadia Community College, 2020).

6 Jodi Melamed, *Racial Capitalism* (Minneapolis: University of Minnesota Press, 2015), 76–85.

7 Manuela Picq, "Indigenous Politics of Resistance: An Introduction," *New Diversities* 19, no. 2 (2017): 2, newdiversities.mmg.mpg.de/wp-content/uploads/2018/02/2017 _19-02_01_Introduction.pdf.

8 Camille Barton, Psychedelic Seminars, June 20, 2020, www.psychsems.com/episodes /history-drug-war-colonization-racism.

9 Avinash Tharoor, "Report: Global Drug Trafficking Market Worth Half a Trillion Dollars," Talking Drugs, April 21, 2017, www.talkingdrugs.org/report-global -illegal-drug-trade-valued-at-around-half-a-trillion-dollars.

10 Drug Policy Alliance, "Race and the Drug War," https://drugpolicy.org/issues /race-and-drug-war.

11 "1648–1768 – The First Written Reports of Ayahuasca Made by Jesuit Missionaries," Kahpi: The Ayahuasca Hub, 2020, https://ayahuasca-timeline.kahpi.net /ayahuasca-first-reports-jesuit-missionaries/.

12 Rosalía Acosta López, Inti Garcia Flores, and Sarai Piña Alcántara, "Mazatec Perspectives on the Globalization of Psilocybin Mushrooms," Chacruna Institute, May 6, 2020, https://chacruna.net/mazatec-perspectives-on-the-globalization-of -psilocybin-mushrooms/.

13 Jonathon Dickinson, "Iboga Root: Dynamics of Iboga's African Origins and Modern Medical Use," *Journal of the American Botanical Council,* no. 109 (Spring 2016): www.herbalgram.org/resources/herbalgram/issues/109/table-of-contents /hg109-feat-iboga/.

14 Nick Estes, *Our History Is the Future: Standing Rock Versus the Dakota Access Pipeline, and the Long Tradition of Indigenous Resistance* (Brooklyn, NY: Verso Books, 2019), 18.

15 Alexander Dawson, *The Peyote Effect* (Berkeley, CA: University of California Press, 2018).

16 Dawson, *The Peyote Effect,* 17.

17 Kevin Feeney, *Peyote & the Native American Church: An Ethnobotanical Study at the Intersection of Religion, Medicine, Market Exchange, and Law,* PhD Diss., Washington State University, 2016.

18 Diana Negrin, "Colonial Shadows in the Psychedelic Renaissance," Chacruna Institute, June 9, 2020, https://chacruna.net/colonial-shadows-in-the-psychedelic -renaissance/.

19 "1879–1912—Ayahuasca Use Spread as the Rubber Boom Decimated Natives," Kahpi: The Ayahuasca Hub, 2020, https://ayahuasca-timeline.kahpi.net/rubber-boom -ayahuasca-indigenous/.

20 Michael Taussig, *Shamanism, Colonialism, and the Wild Man: A Study in Terror and Healing* (Chicago: University of Chicago Press, 1987); "1987—Shamanism, Colonialism, and the Wild Man Is Published," Kahpi: The Ayahuasca Hub, 2020, https://ayahuasca-timeline.kahpi.net/shamanism-colonialism-yage-taussig/.

21 Maestra Vicky Corisepa, "Don't Forget Us Native People Behind the Ayahuasca," Kahpi: The Ayahuasca Hub, November 23, 2019, https://kahpi.net/indigenous-amazonian-native-people-ayahuasca/.

22 Maestro Pedro Tangoa López, "The Dangers of the Ayahuasca Tourism Boom," Kahpi: The Ayahuasca Hub, January 22, 2020, https://kahpi.net/ayahuasca-tourism-boom-pedro-tangoa-lopez/.

23 Max Opray, "Tourist Boom for Ayahuasca a Mixed Blessing for Amazon," *The Guardian,* January 24, 2017, www.theguardian.com/sustainable-business/2017/jan/24/tourist-boom-peru-ayahuasca-drink-amazon-spirituality-healing.

24 "1986–2003—Ayahuasca Is Patented in the US," Kahpi: The Ayahuasca Hub, 2020, https://ayahuasca-timeline.kahpi.net/ayahuasca-us-patent-trademark/.

25 Jeffrey L. Fox, "Bioprospectors Blocked," *Nature Biotechnology* 17, no. 411, (May 1999): https://doi.org/10.1038/8553.

26 Jocelyn Bosse, (@JocelynBosse), "Let's talk about the infamous plant patent for ayahuasca . . .," Twitter, June 21, 2021, https://twitter.com/JocelynBosse/status/1406944990815830017.

27 "In the Declaration of Yarinacocha, Shipibo Healers Organize to Resist Spiritual Extractivism," The Shipibo Conibo Center of New York, Amazon Watch, September 7, 2018, https://amazonwatch.org/news/2018/0907-in-the-declaration-of-yarinacocha-shipibo-healers-organize-to-resist-spiritual-extractivism.

28 "Historias y Memorias Mazatecas," Fungi Foundation, ffungi.org/en/mazatecas.

29 "Preamble to Trail of Broken Treaties 20-Point Position Paper," American Indian Movement Grand Governing Council, https://aimovement.org/ggc/trailofbrokentreaties.html.

30 Picq, "Indigenous Politics of Resistance," 2; Leanne Betasamosake Simpson, *As We Have Always Done: Indigenous Freedom Through Radical Resurgence* (Minneapolis: University of Minnesota Press, 2017).

31 "Fact Sheet: Missing and Murdered Aboriginal Women and Girls," Native Women's Association of Canada, www.nwac.ca/assets-knowledge-centre/Fact_Sheet_Missing_and_Murdered_Aboriginal_Women_and_Girls.pdf.

32 Native Women's Association of Canada, "Reclaiming Power and Place," www.mmiwg-ffada.ca/final-report.

33 The Red Nation, "The Red Nation Manifesto," 9, https://therednationdotorg.files.wordpress.com/2015/03/trn-pamphlet-manifesto-edits.pdf.

34 "About," Protect the Peaks, https://protectthepeaks.org/about/.

35 "Unist'ot'en Healing Centre," UnistotenCamp, video, 3:23, December 5, 2018, https://www.youtube.com/watch?v=MQ2fr0ot6CQ.

36 M. Ito, and H. Nichols, "Kū Kia'i Mauna: Mauna Kea, Protecting the Sacred, and the Thirty Meter Telescope," University of Virginia, 2021, https://religionlab.virginia.edu/projects/ku-kia%CA%BBi-mauna-mauna-kea-protecting-the-sacred-and-the-thirty-meter-telescope/.

37 J. Valle Ayuque and S. Ortega, "The Tragic Death of Peruvian Indigenous Healer Olivia Arévalo," Open Democracy, May 11, 2018, www.opendemocracy.net/en/democraciaabierta/tragic-death-of-indigenous-healer-olivia-ar-v/.

38 L. Salazar-López, "Inspiration, Healing, and Resistance from Amazonian Women Defenders," Amazon Watch, March 28, 2022, https://amazonwatch.org/news /2022/0328-inspiration-healing-and-resistance-from-amazonian-women-defenders.

39 "Public Manifesto of the Women of the Indigenous Nationalities of the Ecuadorian Amazon," Amazon Watch, March 8, 2022, https://amazonwatch.org/assets/files /2022-03-08-confenaie-public-manifesto-eng.pdf.

40 "What Does Land Restitution Mean and How Does It Relate to the Land Back Movement?" Community-Based Global Learning Collaborative, www.cbglcollab.org/what -does-land-restitution-mean.

41 Land Back, Landback.org; NDN Collective, https://ndncollective.org.

42 Glenn Sean Coulthard, *Red Skin, White Masks: Rejecting the Colonial Politics of Recognition* (Minneapolis: University of Minnesota Press, 2014), 31.

43 Resource Generation, "Land Reparations & Indigenous Solidarity Toolkit," https:// resourcegeneration.org/land-reparations-indigenous-solidarity-action-guide/.

44 Macarena Gómez-Barris, *The Extractive Zone: Social Ecologies and Decolonial Perspectives* (Raleigh, NC: Duke University Press, 2017), xix.

45 Bonaventure Soh Bejeng Ndikung, "Where Do We Go from Here: For They Shall Be Heard," *Frieze* 199 (October 28, 2018).

46 M. Daut, "When France Extorted Haiti—The Greatest Heist in History," *The Conversation,* June 30, 2020, https://theconversation.com/when-france-extorted-haiti -the-greatest-heist-in-history-137949.

47 Greg Rosalsky, "The Greatest Heist in History': How Haiti Was Forced to Pay Reparations for Freedom," NPR, October 5, 2021, https://www.npr.org/sections/money /2021/10/05/1042518732/-the-greatest-heist-in-history-how-haiti-was-forced -to-pay-reparations-for-freed.

48 Eve Tuck and K. Wayne Yang, "Decolonization Is Not a Metaphor," *Decolonization: Indigeneity, Education & Society* 1, no. 1 (2012): 21.

Chapter 12: Reciprocity

1 LaDonna Harris and Jacqueline Wasilewski, "Indigeneity: An Alternative Worldview," *Systems Research and Behavioral Science* 21, no. 5 (October 11, 2004): 492–93, www.humiliationstudies.org/documents/WasilewskiIndigeneity.pdf.

2 "How to Come Correct," Sogorea Te' Land Trust, May 6, 2021, https://sogoreate -landtrust.org/how-to-come-correct/.

3 Leanne Simpson, "Dancing the World into Being," interview by Naomi Klein, *Yes!,* March 6, 2013, www.yesmagazine.org/social-justice/2013/03/06/dancing-the-world -into-being-a-conversation-with-idle-no-more-leanne-simpson.

4 Lina D. Dostilio et al., "Reciprocity: Saying What We Mean and Meaning What We Say," *Michigan Journal of Community Service Learning* 19, no. 1 (Fall 2012): 26, http://hdl.handle.net/2027/spo.3239521.0019.102.

5 Harris and Wasilewski, "Indigeneity."

6 Eduardo Schenberg and Konstantin Gerber, "Overcoming Epistemic Injustices in the Biomedical Study of Ayahuasca: Towards Ethical and Sustainable Regulation," *Transcultural Psychiatry* 59, no. 5 (October 2022).

7 Schenberg and Gerber, "Ayahuasca."

8 J. Gray, et al., "Protecting the Sacred Tree: Conceptualizing Spiritual Abuse Against Native American Elders," *Psychology of Religion and Spirituality* 13, no. 2 (2018): 204–11.

9 Gómez-Barris, Preface, in *The Extractive Zone,* xiii–xx.

10	Anna Lutkajtis, "Lost Saints: Desacralization, Spiritual Abuse, and Magic Mushrooms," *Fieldwork in Religion* 14, no. 2 (March 31, 2020): 124.

11	Lutkajtis, "Lost Saints," 118–39.

12	M. R. Duke, "Gordon Wasson's Disembodied Eye: Genre, Representation and the Dialectics of Subjectivity in Huautla de Jiménez, Mexico," (PhD Diss., University of Texas, 1996), 119.

13	Lutkajtis, "Lost Saints," 137; Duke, "Wasson," 269; P. Faudree, "Tales from the Land of Magic Plants: Textual Ideologies and Fetishes of Indigeneity in Mexico's Sierra Mazateca," *Comparative Studies in Society and History* 57, no. 3, 2015: 838–69; Inti Flores, "On Maria Sabina and the Mazatec Heritage with Inti and Paula," *The Psychedologist,* July 2018.

14	William Adams and Martin Mulligan, "Nature and the Colonial Mind," in *Decolonizing Nature: Strategies for Conservation in a Post-Colonial Era* (London: Taylor & Francis, 2012), 16–44.

15	Schenberg and Gerber, "Ayahuasca," 616.

16	Alexander Dawson, *The Peyote Effect* (Berkeley, CA: University of California Press, 2018) 28–29.

17	Simpson and Klein, "Dancing the World into Being."

18	Ruth Goldstein, "Ethnobotanies of Refusal: Methodologies in Respecting Plant(ed)–Human Resistance," *Anthropology Today* 35, no. 2 (April 1, 2019): 21.

19	K. Gerber, I. Flores, A. Ruiz, I. Ali, N. Ginsberg and E. Schenberg, "Ethical Concerns About Psilocybin Intellectual Property," *ACS Pharmacology & Translational Science* 4, no. 2 (January 2021): 576.

20	Maestra Vicky Corisepa, "Don't Forget Us Native People Behind the Ayahuasca," Kahpi: The Ayahuasca Hub, November 23, 2019, https://kahpi.net/indigenous -amazonian-native-people-ayahuasca/.

21	Nick Estes, "Native Liberation: The Way Forward," *The Red Nation*, August 17, 2016, https://therednation.org/native-liberation-the-way-forward/.

22	Linda Tuhiwai Smith, *Decolonizing Methodologies: Research and Indigenous Peoples* (London: Zed Books, 1999), 118–20.

23	Mohr, "Psychedelic Extractivism."

24	Gómez-Barris, "Introduction: Submerged Perspectives," in *The Extractive Zone,* 1–16.

25	Gómez-Barris, "Submerged Perspectives," xix.

26	Raymond Murphy, "Rationalization Under the Premise of Plasticity," in *Rationality and Nature: A Sociological Inquiry into a Changing Relationship* (London: Routledge, 1994), 3–26.

27	Val Plumwood, "Decolonizing Relationships with Nature," in *Decolonizing Nature*, 52.

28	Resmaa Menakem, *My Grandmother's Hands: Racialized Trauma and the Pathway to Mending Our Hearts and Bodies* (Las Vegas: Central Recovery Press, 2017).

29	Joy Harjo, *The Spiral of Memory* (Ann Arbor: University of Michigan Press, 2021), 93.

30	Harris and Wasilewski, "Indigeneity."

31	"In the Declaration of Yarinacocha, Shipibo Healers Organize to Resist Spiritual Extractivism," Shipibo Conibo Center of New York, Amazon Watch, September 7, 2018, https://amazonwatch.org/news/2018/0907-in-the-declaration-of-yarinacocha -shipibo-healers-organize-to-resist-spiritual-extractivism.

32	"Pronouncement of the Shipibo-Konibo-Xetebo Nation on the Globalization of Ayahuasca," Asociación de Onanyabo Médicos Ancestrales Shipibo Kobino, 2019.

33	Indigenous Peyote Conservation Initiative (IPCI), www.ipci.life.

Chapter 13: Hope

1 Brian Sonenstein and Kim Wilson, "Hope Is a Discipline feat. Mariame Kaba," January 5, 2018, in *Beyond Prisons*, podcast, 54:30, www.beyond-prisons.com/home /hope-is-a-discipline-feat-mariame-kaba.

2 "Hope Is a Discipline: Mariame Kaba on Dismantling the Carceral State," March 17, 2021, in *Intercepted*, podcast, 35:44, https://theintercept.com/2021/03/17 /intercepted-mariame-kaba-abolitionist-organizing/.

3 adrienne maree brown, *Pleasure Activism* (Chico, CA: AK Press, 2019), 437.

4 Bill Brennan, "The Revolution Will Not Be Psychologized: Psychedelics' Potential for Systemic Change," Chacruna Institute, July 3, 2020, https://chacruna.net/the -revolution-will-not-be-psychologized-psychedelics-potential-for-systemic -change/.

5 Kelly Hayes and Mariame Kaba, *Let This Radicalize You: Organizing and the Revolution of Reciprocal Care* (Chicago: Haymarket Books, 2023).

BIBLIOGRAPHY

2012 Green Dot Team Cadre: Bayou, Blackswan, and Duneydan. "Green Dot Advanced Ranger Training Manual." 2012. rangers.burningman.org/wp-content/uploads/GD -manual-2012.pdf.

Adams, William and Martin Mulligan. "Nature and the Colonial Mind." In *Decolonizing Nature: Strategies for Conservation in a Post-Colonial Era,* 16–44. London: Taylor & Francis, 2012.

Amazon Watch. "Public Manifesto of the Women of the Indigenous Nationalities of the Ecuadorian Amazon." 2022. https://amazonwatch.org/assets/files/2022-03-08 -confenaie-public-manifesto-eng.pdf.

"American Indian Movement: Grand Governing Council." Aimovement.org.

"Anti-Oppression Training & Resources Alliance." AORTA.Coop.

Barnard Center for Research on Women. "What Is Transformative Justice?" YouTube, March 11, 2020. www.youtube.com/watch?v=U-_BOFz5TXo.

Bosse, Jocelyn (@JocelynBosse). "Let's talk about the infamous plant patent for ayahuasca. . . ." Twitter, June 21, 2021. https://twitter.com/JocelynBosse/status /1406944990815830017.

Brennan, Bill. "The Revolution Will Not Be Psychologized: Psychedelics' Potential for Systemic Change." Chacruna Institute, July 3, 2020. https://chacruna.net/the -revolution-will-not-be-psychologized-psychedelics-potential-for-systemic-change/.

brown, adrienne maree. *Emergent Strategy.* Chico, CA: AK Press, 2017.

———. *Pleasure Activism.* Chico, CA: AK Press, 2019.

———. *We Will Not Cancel Us.* Chico, CA: AK Press, 2020.

Cheng Thom, Kai. *I Hope We Choose Love.* Vancouver, BC: Arsenal Pulp Press, 2019.

Cole, S., J. Capitanio, K. Chun, J. Arevalo, J. Ma, and J. Cacioppo. "Myeloid Differentiation Architecture of Leukocyte Transcriptome Dynamics in Perceived Social Isolation." *Proceedings of the National Academy of Sciences of the United States of America* 112, no. 49 (November 23, 2015): 15142–7. https://pubmed.ncbi.nlm.nih.gov/26598672.

Community-Based Global Learning Collaborative. "What Does Land Restitution Mean and How Does It Relate to the Land Back Movement?" www.cbglcollab.org /what-does-land-restitution-mean.

Corisepa, Maestra Vicky. "Don't Forget Us Native People Behind the Ayahuasca." Kahpi: The Ayahuasca Hub, November 23, 2019. https://kahpi.net/indigenous-amazonian -native-people-ayahuasca/.

Coulthard, Glenn Sean. *Red Skin, White Masks: Rejecting the Colonial Politics of Recognition.* Minneapolis: University of Minnesota Press, 2014.

Cuentas, Claudia. "About: Claudia Cuentas." Claudiacuentas.com.

Daut, M. "When France Extorted Haiti—The Greatest Heist in History." The Conversation. June 30, 2020. https://theconversation.com/when-france-extorted-haiti-the-greatest -heist-in-history-137949.

Dawson, Alexander. *The Peyote Effect.* Berkeley, CA: University of California Press, 2018.

Des Jarlais, D. "Harm Reduction in the USA: The Research Perspective and an Archive to David Purchase." *Harm Reduction Journal* 14, no. 51 (2017).

Dickinson, J. "Iboga Root: Dynamics of Iboga's African Origins and Modern Medical Use." *The Journal of the American Botanical Council,* no. 109, (Spring 2016): 48–57.

www.herbalgram.org/resources/herbalgram/issues/109/table-of-contents/hg109
-feat-iboga/.

Dostilio, L., et al. "Reciprocity: Saying What We Mean and Meaning What We Say."
Michigan Journal of Community Service Learning 19, no. 1 (Fall 2012): 17–32. http://
hdl.handle.net/2027/spo.3239521.0019.102.

Drug Policy Alliance. "Race and the Drug War." https://drugpolicy.org/issues/race-and
-drug-war.

Duckworth, Sylvia. "Wheel of Power and Privilege" (adapted from https://ccrweb.ca
/en/power-wheel-update). www.rwuc.org/wp-content/uploads/2021/09/wheel.pdf.

Duke, M. R. "Gordon Wasson's Disembodied Eye: Genre, Representation and the Dia-
lectics of Subjectivity in Huautla de Jiménez, Mexico." PhD Diss., University of
Texas, 1996.

Estes, Nick. *Our History Is the Future: Standing Rock Versus the Dakota Access Pipeline,
and the Long Tradition of Indigenous Resistance.* New York: Verso Books, 2019.

Faudree, P. "Tales from the Land of Magic Plants: Textual Ideologies and Fetishes of Indigeneity in Mexico's Sierra Mazateca." *Comparative Studies in Society and History* 57,
no. 3 (2015): 838–69.

Feeney, K. "Peyote & the Native American Church: An Ethnobotanical Study at the
Intersection of Religion, Medicine, Market Exchange, and Law." PhD Diss., Washington State University, 2016.

Flores, Inti García. "On María Sabina and the Mazatec Heritage with Inti and Paula." *The
Psychedelogist.* July 2018.

Fox, J. "Bioprospectors Blocked." *Nature Biotechnology* 17, no. 411 (May 1999): https://
doi.org/10.1038/8553.

Friedwoman, Leia. "How the Psychedelic Community Should Respond to Sexual
Abuse." Lucid News. October 29, 2021, www.lucid.news/how-the-psychedelic
-community-should-respond-to-sexual-abuse/.

Frontline. "Opium Throughout History." www.pbs.org/wgbh/pages/frontline/shows
/heroin/etc/history.html.

Fungi Foundation. "Historias Y Memorias Mazatecas." www.ffungi.org/en/mazatecas.

Gerber, K., I. Flores, A. Ruiz, I. Ali, N. Ginsberg, and E. Schenberg. "Ethical Concerns
About Psilocybin Intellectual Property." *ACS Pharmacology & Translational Science*
4, no. 2 (January 2021): 573–77.

Goldstein, R. "Ethnobotanies of Refusal: Methodologies in Respecting Plant(ed)-Human
Resistance." *Anthropology Today* 35, no. 2 (April 1, 2019): 18–22.

Gómez-Barris, Macarena. "Preface." In *The Extractive Zone: Social Ecologies and Decolonial Perspectives,* xiii–xx. Raleigh, NC: Duke University Press, 2017.

———. "Introduction: Submerged Perspectives." In *The Extractive Zone: Social Ecologies and Decolonial Perspectives,* 1–16. Raleigh, NC: Duke University Press, 2017.

Gray, J., et al. "Protecting the Sacred Tree: Conceptualizing Spiritual Abuse Against
Native American Elders." *Psychology of Religion and Spirituality* 13, no. 2 (2018): 204–11.

Haines, Staci K. *The Politics of Trauma.* Berkeley, CA: North Atlantic Books, 2019.

Harris, LaDonna and Jacqueline Wasilewski. "Indigeneity: An Alternative Worldview,"
Systems Research and Behavioral Science 21, no. 5 (October 11, 2004): 489–503. www
.humiliationstudies.org/documents/WasilewskiIndigeneity.pdf.

"Hope Is a Discipline: Mariame Kaba on Dismantling the Carceral State." March 17, 2021.
In *Intercepted,* podcast, 35:44. https://theintercept.com/2021/03/17/intercepted
-mariame-kaba-abolitionist-organizing/.

"In the Declaration of Yarinacocha, Shipibo Healers Organize to Resist Spiritual Extractivism." The Shipibo Conibo Center of New York, Amazon Watch. September 7, 2018.

https://amazonwatch.org/news/2018/0907-in-the-declaration-of-yarinacocha
-shipibo-healers-organize-to-resist-spiritual-extractivism.

Ito, M. and H. Nichols. "Kū Kiaʻi Mauna: Mauna Kea, Protecting the Sacred, and the Thirty Meter Telescope." University of Virginia, 2021. https://religionlab.virginia
.edu/projects/ku-kia%CA%BBi-mauna-mauna-kea-protecting-the-sacred-and-the
-thirty-meter-telescope/.

Jacanimijoy, A. "Open Letter to the Congress of the United States." April 6, 1998.

C. G. Jung. *Psychology and Religion: West and East (The Collected Works of C. G. Jung, Vol. 11)*. Princeton, NJ: Princeton University Press, 1938.

Kaba, Mariame. *We Do This Till We Free Us*. Chicago: Haymarket Books, 2021.

Kaba, Mariame and Shira Hassan. *Fumbling Towards Repair*. Project NIA, 2019.

Kendi, Ibram X. *Stamped from the Beginning*. New York: Bold Type Books, 2016.

Kimmerer, Robin Wall. "Honorable Harvest: Lessons from an Indigenous Tradition of Giving Thanks." *Yes!* November 26, 2015. www.yesmagazine.org/issue
/good-health/2015/11/26/the-honorable-harvest-lessons-from-an-indigenous
-tradition-of-giving-thanks.

LandBack. Landback.org.

López, Rosalía Acosta, Inti García Flores, and Sarai Piña Alcántara. "Mazatec Perspectives on the Globalization of Psilocybin Mushrooms." Chacruna Institute, May 6, 2020. https://
chacruna.net/mazatec-perspectives-on-the-globalization-of-psilocybin-mushrooms/.

Lutkajtis, Anna. "Lost Saints: Desacralization, Spiritual Abuse, and Magic Mushrooms." *Fieldwork in Religion* 14, no. 2 (March 31, 2020): 118–39.

McLane, Hannah and Emma Knighton. "Narcissism in the Psychedelic Ecosystem." Chacruna Institute, September 14, 2022. www.crowdcast.io/e/narcissism-in-the/register.

Melamed, J. *Racial Capitalism*. Minneapolis: University of Minnesota Press, 2015.

Mohr, Juliette. Juliette Mohr. juliettemohr.digital.

———. "Psychedelic Extractivism: Distilling Indigeneity into Exchange Value." 2021.
https://www.juliettemohr.digital/post/psychedelic-extractivism.

Native Women's Association of Canada. "Fact Sheet: Missing and Murdered Aboriginal Women and Girls." NWAC. www.nwac.ca/assets-knowledge-centre/Fact_Sheet
_Missing_and_Murdered_Aboriginal_Women_and_Girls.pdf.

———. "Written Brief Submitted to the House of Commons Standing Committee on the Status of Women for Its Study on Intimate Partner and Domestic Violence in Canada,"
1. Parliament of Canada. www.ourcommons.ca/Content/Committee/441/FEWO
/Brief/BR11685394/br-external/NativeWomensAssociationOfCanada-e.pdf.

Negrin, Diana. "Colonial Shadows in the Psychedelic Renaissance." Chacruna Institute, June 9, 2020. https://chacruna.net/colonial-shadows-in-the-psychedelic-renaissance/.

Oak, Annie. "Manual of Best Practices for Radical Risk Reduction." Women's Visionary Council, November 2018. https://visionarycongress.org/articles/wvc-articles
/manual-radical-risk-reduction/.

———. *The Manual of Psychedelic Support: A Practical Guide to Establishing and Facilitating Care Services at Music Festivals and Other Events*, 2nd ed. San Jose, CA: Multidisciplinary Association for Psychedelic Studies (MAPS), 2017. https://maps.org
/product/manual-of-psychedelic-support/.

Opray, Max. "Tourist Boom for Ayahuasca a Mixed Blessing for Amazon." *The Guardian*, January 24, 2017. www.theguardian.com/sustainable-business/2017/jan/24
/tourist-boom-peru-ayahuasca-drink-amazon-spirituality-healing.

Picq, Manuela. "Indigenous Politics of Resistance: An Introduction." *New Diversities* 19, no. 2 (2017): 1–6. newdiversities.mmg.mpg.de/wp-content/uploads/2018/02/2017
_19-02_01_Introduction.pdf.

Piepzna-Samarasinha, L. *Beyond Survival.* Chico, CA: AK Press, 2020.

"Pronouncement of the Shipibo-Konibo-Xetebo Nation on the Globalization of Aya-huasca." Asociación de Onanyabo Médicos Ancestrales Shipibo Konibo, 2019.

Protect the Peaks. "About." https://protectthepeaks.org/about/.

The Psychedologist. "Consciousness—Positivity—Radio." thepsychedologist.com.

The Red Nation. "The Red Nation Manifesto." https://therednationdotorg.files.word press.com/2015/03/trn-pamphlet-manifesto-edits.pdf.

Resource Generation. "Land Reparations & Indigenous Solidarity Toolkit." https:// resourcegeneration.org/land-reparations-indigenous-solidarity-action-guide/.

Reynolds, V. "An Ethical Stance for Justice-Doing in Community Work and Therapy." *Journal of Systemic Therapies* 31, no. 4 (2012): 18–33.

Rivera, Justice and Shaan Lashun. *Towards Bodily Autonomy* (Self-published, 2023).

Robinson, Cedric. *Black Marxism: The Making of the Black Radical Tradition.* Raleigh, NC: University of North Carolina Press, 1983.

Rosalsky, Greg. "'The Greatest Heist in History': How Haiti Was Forced to Pay Repa-rations for Freedom." NPR, October 5, 2021. https://www.npr.org/sections/money /2021/10/05/1042518732/-the-greatest-heist-in-history-how-haiti-was-forced-to -pay-reparations-for-freed.

Salazar-López, L. "Inspiration, Healing, and Resistance from Amazonian Women Defend-ers." Amazon Watch, March 28, 2022. https://amazonwatch.org/news/2022/0328 -inspiration-healing-and-resistance-from-amazonian-women-defenders.

Saneda, Tori and Michelle Field. "Cultural Anthropology: Legacy of Colonialism." Cas-cadia Community College, 2020.

Schenberg, Eduardo and Konstantin Gerber. "Overcoming Epistemic Injustices in the Biomedical Study of Ayahuasca: Towards Ethical and Sustainable Regulation." *Transcultural Psychiatry* 59, no. 5 (October 2022): 611–24.

Shiva, Vandana. *Biopiracy: The Plunder of Nature and Knowledge.* East Sussex, UK: Green Books in Association with the Gaia Foundation, 1998.

Simpson, Leanne. "Dancing the World into Being." Interview by Naomi Klein. *Yes!,* March 6, 2013. www.yesmagazine.org/social-justice/2013/03/06/dancing-the-world -into-being-a-conversation-with-idle-no-more-leanne-simpson.

Smith, Linda Tuhiwai. *Decolonizing Methodologies: Research and Indigenous Peoples.* London: Zed Books, 1999.

Sogorea Te' Land Trust. "How to Come Correct." May 6, 2021. https://sogoreate-landtrust .org/how-to-come-correct/.

Soh Bejeng Ndikung, Bonaventure. "Where Do We Go from Here: For They Shall Be Heard." *Frieze* no. 199, October 28, 2018.

Sonenstein, Brian and Kim Wilson. "Hope Is a Discipline feat. Mariame Kaba." January 5, 2018. In *Beyond Prison,* podcast, 54:30. https://www.beyond-prisons.com/home /hope-is-a-discipline-feat-mariame-kaba.

Suarez, Cyndi. *The Power Manual,* 26. British Columbia, Canada: New Society Publish-ers, 2018.

Taylor, Kylea. *The Ethics of Caring.* Santa Cruz, CA: Hanford Mead, 1995.

Tharoor, Avinash. "Report: Global Drug Trafficking Market Worth Half a Trillion Dollars." Talking Drugs, April 21, 2017. www.talkingdrugs.org/report-global-illegal-drug-trade -valued-at-around-half-a-trillion-dollars.

Tuck, Eve and K. Wayne Yang. "Decolonization Is Not a Metaphor." *Decolonization: Indi-geneity, Education & Society* 1, no. 1 (2012): 1–40.

"Unist'ot'en Healing Centre." UnistotenCamp. December 5, 2018. YouTube, video, 3:23. https://www.youtube.com/watch?v=MQ2fr0ot6CQ.

Washington, Hanifa Nayo. "About: Hanifa Nayo Washington." Hands of Hanifa, handsof hanifa.com.

White, Joshua and Juliana Mulligan. "Questions to Discuss with a Prospective Psychedelic Facilitator." Fireside Project, June 30, 2022. https://firesideproject.medium.com /questions-to-discuss-with-a-prospective-psychedelic-facilitator-2e36bc932040.

Wikipedia. "Foursquare Church," en.wikipedia.org/wiki/Foursquare_Church.

Women's Visionary Congress. "20 Safety Tips for Those Participating in Ceremonies That Use Psychoactive Substances." December 2014. https://visionarycongress.org /articles/wvc-articles/safety-tips-r3/.

Women's Visionary Council. "Mission and Work." https://visionarycongress.org/about /about-wvc/.

Women's Visionary Congress. "What Elders Offer to Psychedelic Communities." February 2023. https://visionarycongress.org/articles/wvc-articles/what-elders-offer-to -psychedelic-communities-r9/.

INDEX

ABOUT THE AUTHOR

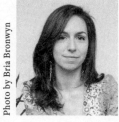

Photo by Bria Bronwyn

Rebecca Martinez is a Xicana writer, community organizer, and social entrepreneur born and living on Chinook land known as Portland, Oregon. Martinez's work explores the intersections between collective healing, systems design, and expanded states of consciousness. She is a student of transformative justice, Emergent Strategy, Somatic Abolitionism, and regenerative landscape design. She is the founder and executive director of Alma Institute, a nonprofit educational institution that equips students from marginalized communities to become legal psychedelic facilitators. She was a cocreator of the *Fruiting Bodies* podcast and a staff member of the Measure 109 campaign that produced the Psilocybin Services Act, the first-ever state program to provide community-based, legal access to psilocybin services. Martinez has served as an advisor to the National Psychedelics Association, the American Psychedelic Practitioners Association, and the Plant Medicine Healing Alliance. She is a voice on psychedelic justice and has been featured in NPR, *Business Insider,* STAT News, Lucid News, *Psychedelics Today,* and several documentaries.

ABOUT NORTH ATLANTIC BOOKS

North Atlantic Books (NAB) is an independent, nonprofit publisher committed to a bold exploration of the relationships between mind, body, spirit, and nature. Founded in 1974, NAB aims to nurture a holistic view of the arts, sciences, humanities, and healing. To make a donation or to learn more about our books, authors, events, and newsletter, please visit www.northatlanticbooks.com.